WOW. TH/

Fred oiver

DEALING WITH VISION LOSS

by
Fred Olver

authorHOUSE

AuthorHouse™
1663 Liberty Drive, Suite 200
Bloomington, IN 47403
www.authorhouse.com
Phone: 1-800-839-8640

© *2007 Fred Olver. All rights reserved.*

No part of this book may be reproduced, stored in a retrieval system, or
transmitted by any means without the written permission of the author.

First published by AuthorHouse 8/8/2007

ISBN: 978-1-4343-1493-2 (sc)

Printed in the United States of America
Bloomington, Indiana

This book is printed on acid-free paper.

You may not copy or distribute this book without the expressed written permission of the
author. This book is for your use only. If you have questions or comments, please send
them by e-mail, in Braille, or on tape to:

FRED OLVER
P.O. Box 43006
Maplewood, MO 63143
goodfolks@charter.net

This book is available in alternative formats including audio recording and digital
download through the website:
http://www.dealingwithvisionloss.com

This author is not responsible for any incorrect information such as addresses, phone
numbers and web page addresses. As of the writing of this book they were verified as
much as possible.

ACKNOWLEDGEMENTS

First of all, this book is dedicated to my daughter, Margaret, because of her seemingly ever-lasting faith in me as a father and a single parent for the last twelve years.

Secondly, I would like to acknowledge my parents and their faith in me as an individual. When my dad gave me a motorcycle as a gift for graduating from high school, he believed I would be able to ride it. When I wanted to attend public school, my senior year of high school, my parents supported me, even though I contacted the school before asking them how they felt about it or if it was okay to do so.

Next I wish to thank Peggy Magathan, a lady I met in Charleston, South Carolina many years ago. She told me I had a book in me, and although I agreed with her, I never thought it would happen because I thought I needed to be in a particular place or have a certain attitude. Turns out, all I needed to do was sit down and start writing.

I could not send this book to the publisher without acknowledging the work of my editor. She is truly a person whom I am proud to call my friend.
She doesn't treat me like a blind person; she treats me as if blindness is just one part of who I am. She brings things to my attention that I otherwise might miss, asking the best of me, and encouraging me to give my best in my writing and in my observations within these pages. When she made

suggestions about the book, I knew it was for the benefit of the reader and I made sure to listen closely. Thank you, Donnagail.

And lastly this book is dedicated to the lady who introduced me to "BRAILLE KISSES".

I could think of many other people to acknowledge, thank or mention, but I think this book is the sum of having met so many diverse and wonderful people. It is the culmination of their beliefs, their views, their comments to me, but mostly I suppose, my observations which have brought me to this point in my life. I hope you will read this book from cover to cover and I hope you gain some sense of security, some sense of ability rather than disability from its contents.

Contents

FORWARD ix
    Definitions. x
    A Further Note xiv
    A Bit Of History xv

FAMILY MEMBERS AND VISION LOSS 1
    Adjusting to Vision Loss. 3
    Acceptance Of Vision Loss. 11
    Dealing With A Blind Person For The First Time. 13
    The Reality Of Blindness 17
    An Introduction To Blindness. 21

DIMINISHED VISION AND YOU 27
    Encountering Diminished Vision 29
    Living Independently In The 21st Century. 35
    The Rehabilitation Process And Beyond 42
    Computers And You 45
    Orienting Yourself To A Table 48
    Some Other Hints 50
    Environmental Modification. 54
    Guiding And Being Guided 54
    Orientation And Mobility For Adults 57
    Deciding To Use A Cane. 60
    You And Dog Guides 61
    Barriers And Overcoming Them. 63
    Transitions. 73

KIDS AND BLINDNESS 75
    Determining Vision Loss 77
    Braille And Other Communications Skills 78
    Orientation And Mobility For Kids. 81
    Public School Or School For The Blind 86
    Summer Camps And Your Child. 89
    Finishing Touches. 90

RESOURCES AND CATALOGS 97

AN ASSAULT ON YOUR SENSES 165

vii

FORWARD

Why am I writing this book? First off, I have been told by a number of individuals that there is a book in me. I am as of this writing, 54 years old and endeavoring to start a new career. I have worked at several jobs in my life including: tele-marketing, factory work, functioned as a library aide, taught at rehabilitation agencies both state and private, and as well, been on the cutting edge of the development of talking software for use by blind and visually impaired individuals. In fact, when I think about it, I have worked in most areas of the field of blindness. Having worked with both adults and children who were blind or visually impaired as well as my own life experience uniquely qualifies me to speak to you about blindness, it's causes, the effects, both psychological and physical, how to deal with it and the resources that are available throughout the United States and beyond.

Some say I'm lucky because I was born blind, and in fact, they are right. From my experience, I have found that it is much less difficult for me to do things, or to learn how to do things, not having been able to see rather than for an individual who has been able to see. Try looking at it this way; an individual who has been able to make use of their vision up until now has been able to look at that hamburger in the skillet to see how done it actually is, or that shirt to see if it matches the rest of what they are wearing. If they lose their ability to see colors they will need to find some other way to identify colors or determine doneness of food. That's where I would come in. As a Rehabilitation Teacher it was my job to teach people how to do things not using their vision in order to gain information while performing the same tasks. But that's not all. It's not just my experience as a Rehabilitation Teacher which has led me to write this book. Over and over again I have heard from individuals that they had a hard time finding resources for their friend or relative, which would empower them to function as they did before they lost most if not all of their vision.

Everybody and their brother has ideas of what one needs to do in order to adjust to vision loss, where to find the necessary information they need, but I have yet to see a book available anywhere which spells out most of the places where one can go in order to find information about resources or how to deal with vision loss from several different perspectives. This book offers information from three very distinct and different fronts. It provides information for the individual going through the adjustment to having lost most if not all of their vision. It provides information and advice for parents of blind children and also provides a positive presentation for family members of individuals who are experiencing vision loss. I have seen books which attempt to provide information for one of these groups, but not a resource for everyone affected by vision loss. I feel that this book does that and I hope by the time you finish reading it you will too.

DEFINITIONS

When reading this book it's helpful to understand the definitions for some of the special terms you'll encounter.

When I talk about people who are **visually impaired**, I am talking about individuals whose vision is less than 20/20 which for our purposes is considered to be normal vision. Thus, someone with 20/70 or 20/150 visual acuity would be considered visually impaired.

In order to be considered **legally blind**, an individual must have a visual acuity of less than 20/200, that is to say that an individual is considered legally blind if he/she has 10% or less of normal vision. That means what a person with normal vision sees 200 feet away, a person with 10% of normal vision would need to be not more than 20 feet away from that object or sign, in order to see it with the same clarity as you see it at 200 feet. Now, this definition has a second part. If a person has a visual field of less than 20 degrees in width, then they too would be considered legally blind. This means that a person might be able to read the phone book, because they have very good distance vision, but not be able to see more than a couple fingers wide in field. They too, would be considered legally blind.

Sometimes the terms visually impaired and legally blind are used interchangeably, but generally speaking I think that is done so as not to offend individuals who might be considered legally blind but who are just a bit touchy about being considered blind. Thus, some people who are considered to be blind may indeed have some usable vision, while others do not. I myself have some light perception. That is the ability to see some light. Believe it or not, I used to get afraid of the dark when I was a kid just like everyone else. I've gotten over that, but I sometimes wonder whether or not I would be able to get around as well if my eyes needed to be removed.

ACB: American Council of the Blind. One of three organizations of consumers who are blind. They offer job listings on their web site, an internet radio station with four diverse streams of programming, a monthly magazine The Braille Forum to keep members informed about various happenings with regard to legislation, conventions and other information of interest to its members. Within their organization are many divisions and special interests groups involved in everything from employment to computers to parenting, a nationwide group for blind college students and as well a special interest group for parents of blind children.

NFB: National Federation of the Blind. The largest organization of consumers who are blind in the United States boasting a membership of 50,000 members. Publishes a monthly magazine The Braille Monitor for its members which keeps them informed as to legislation concerning people who are blind, advances in technology taking place at the National Center for the Blind and has hundreds of books and materials available for purchase from their web site. Within the organization are some 750 chapters and affiliates in each state, the District of Columbia and Puerto Rico. They offer, via membership, access to more than 50 divisions and special interest groups including the National Association for Blind Students, the National Association of Blind Lawyers, a division for people interested in or participating in equestrian endeavors as well as a special interest group for senior citizens.

BVA Blinded Veterans of America Organization composed of Veterans who have sustained a significant vision loss.

Environmental Cues Information derived from using senses other than vision: hearing, taste, smell and touch.

Rehabilitation Teacher: The person who is mostly responsible for teaching individuals how to function in their homes, within rehabilitation centers, nursing homes or Centers for Independent Living.

O&M instructors sometimes referred to as Orientation and Mobility Instructors: Individuals responsible for teaching someone how to use a cane, and sometimes low vision aids in conjunction with their Orientation and Mobility skills. They also teach individuals route travel, using buses and basically getting around in their community. For example they would teach you how to cross at a light, but not every light in your town or neighborhood. The Orientation thing is explained later.

Low Vision and Low Vision Aids: Low Vision is anyone who has limited but remaining vision. That vision may be of use under certain circumstances, and Low Vision Aids assist an individual in making use of remaining vision. They come in several types:

- hand-held magnifiers used for reading;
- monoculars, usually for improving distance vision in order to be able to read addresses and street signs and

- Closed Circuit TV's (CCTV's) used for magnification of materials to be read and some can be used as monitors for your computer.

Large Print: 14-point type or larger. This book is written in large print. If letters are written in 14-point type or larger they can be mailed free, so long as the envelope is not sealed and "free matter for the blind" is written where the stamp goes.

A FURTHER NOTE

Having read this book through now, most of a hundred times, I do indeed urge you to read it from cover to cover. True, some of the sections have been labeled "for family members" or "kids and blindness, " however unless you read this book entirely you will not learn all you need to know in order to become aware of your needs, the needs of individuals who may be blind or the needs of children who are blind. Blindness is not something I put on in the morning and take off in the evening. I live it every day, and if you are blind, or going to be blind in a matter of time, you too, will need to learn to live it. In order to do that, you need to learn absolutely as much about it as you can, because like it or not, you will become a diplomat, an ambassador of blindness. People are going to ask you all kinds of questions. They will think nothing of asking how you lost your sight. They will expect you to be able to do everything, or nothing. They will look at you and draw conclusions about the entire population of individuals who are blind based on your abilities or seeming lack of them. Just smile, go about your business and keep on livin'. Sometimes you may surprise people, just remember, it's their own ignorance which causes them to be surprised. Sometimes people will treat you very badly. Just remember, they don't know any better. Always remember that blindness is not caused as a result of God's retribution against either you or your family. Sometimes things just happen.

At the back of this book is a wonderful resource list. Places to find large print playing cards, Braille greeting cards, talking software, information about programs for individuals who wish to snow ski and where to purchase magnifiers. You can find out where to get study materials to learn Braille or get your GED at home, where to send your kids for a month in the summer, plan your vacation or where to find large print puzzles or maps of the United States. Last but not least, you may just find answers to the myriad of questions you have: about your feelings, about your fears concerning blindness and your questions about how to get around and how to break the seemingly endless cycle of dependence on others and lack of confidence in yourself. For you this entire book can be a learning process, let it happen.

Fred Olver, a person who is blind, rather than a blind person

A BIT OF HISTORY

When I was growing up, most kids who were considered blind were sent away to schools for the blind, often not less than 50 miles away from their homes. At that time, pre-school programs for blind kids were practically non-existent, and the same was true of finding information for parents who wanted to learn to use Braille in order to be able to assist and communicate with their children who were blind. In fact, there was no mandate to allow blind children to attend public schools, and in most cases they did not. My mother told me that although she wanted to learn Braille, and endeavored to do so, she was told that the only avenue open to her was a Master's degree level course and she could not take that because she was not working on her Master's degree at a nearby university. While involved in a pre-school program for blind children, several of my classmates and I learned to get around at the tender age of from two to six years. Get around, that is without a cane. We were taught to feed ourselves, what different things were like: a spark plug, a frog or what a stack of cards felt like. As well, we were presented with many opportunities to interact with adults. I can't stress enough to those of you who are parents of children who are blind or visually impaired how valuable this information and interaction was to me and is to your child. More about that later.

While at the school for the blind, we were taught the necessary skills to cope with blindness, but not all of them. These included Braille, academics, use of Braille writers and slate and stylus for the kids who used Braille; and large print for the kids who had some usable vision. Either chair caning or piano tuning was taught to most of the boys. If they didn't learn one or the other of these skills, well, because they were blind it was not expected that they would be able to learn a significant job skill anyway. This was true for the most part, until the early to mid-

60's. Don't get me wrong, kids who were blind did go to college, but they were the exception, not the rule, and let's face it, without being able to use a cane, how would they have gotten around their college campuses?

For the girls, home economics was a must, because it was felt that most of them would end up staying at home. For those lucky enough to have been in school from the early to mid-60's and on, cane travel as it was called was taught, mostly to juniors and seniors. The concept of teaching younger children to use a cane was one which was foreign to most mobility instructors, and in fact, Orientation and Mobility instructors were few and far between because Peripatology, the art of using a cane, was not taught to possible instructors on a university level with the exception of being taught to Veterans after World War II, again, until the early 60's.

While at the school for the blind, besides the basic academics, students were encouraged to participate in varsity sports including track and wrestling. As well, there were recreational activities including roller skating, swimming and bowling. I've bowled as high as a 195 and my goal is to bowl a 200 game before I'm finished. Some of us wrote for the school paper which was sent home with report cards to our parents. Some of us learned Morse code and became ham radio operators. Some students upon finishing high school became vending stand and snack bar operators, working in state or federal installations across the country oftentimes making more than enough money to support their families, some as much as $75,000.00 per year.

During the summer between my junior and senior year of high school I attended a college preparatory program in downtown Detroit where I learned to travel safely, with a cane, making use of the city buses, cross at lights and get back to my parents' home on my own. I'll never forget the day I walked in to Burger Chef and asked for a Whopper with a friend, after dodging the traffic on the westbound side of Michigan Avenue in the western suburbs of Detroit.

My senior year of high school was spent in public school. The reason I mention this is because at that time it was not required that public schools provide education to blind students, however with my parents' support I did attend the high school where my older brother had graduated two years earlier. I feel I need to tell you that when I did attend this high school, I had to agree to a couple of things, the first being that if I did not do well in my first semester that I would go back to the school for the blind in order to finish out my senior year. The second was that I was asked to sign a release form which stated that if anything happened to me, for example if I was injured on school property, that the school would not be held responsible. I didn't want to sign it, but felt that if I didn't, I might have to return to the school for the blind for my senior year. Come to think about it, I wonder if that signature was considered legal since I think I was seventeen at the time. Nonetheless, I had a wonderful time in public school. You see I was the first blind student to attend and graduate from that high school and in fact, most if not all of my classmates there had never seen or met a blind person before meeting me. I later went back to do my student teaching there. After finishing high school and receiving a motor cycle from my dad as a graduation present, which I rode proudly while up in the north woods of Michigan and in our backyard, it was on to college.

I was SCARED TO DEATH. I had no idea where I was, or how to get anywhere on campus. Luckily for me, my first semester I had a roommate who was also blind. He and some of his friends were most helpful in assisting me in learning my way to and from my classes. It was easier to learn where my classes were rather than learning the entire campus all at once. That fall was also my first experience with taped books. Up until this time, all of my books had been provided in Braille, but not any more. I had to change my entire method of studying. My books and hand-outs were made available to me, yes, some on tape, but most in print. As a result, readers needed to be found, a method of learning how to study from tapes rather than Braille was learned and schedules integrated in order to get in necessary study time with unknown readers was developed without any idea as to how to do any of this stuff. Nonetheless, some four years later I received my B.S. degree in Secondary Education with my major area of study being Communication Arts and Sciences.

Upon graduation, I stayed in Kalamazoo, Michigan with my roommates until May when I was hired to work as a Library Aide at a library for the blind and physically handicapped in my home town of Wayne, Michigan. This employment lasted more than two years. While working there: speaking to patrons on the phone, assisting with duplication of cassettes, reading tax forms on tape, and receiving other assignments from my supervisor it became quite clear to me that many of the people receiving equipment from the Library for the Blind had no idea how to make use of the equipment nor the ordering process in order to get books. They had been given this equipment. These people were sent print materials. Now remember these folks are recently blind and the only thing they had been told was where the play button was on the cassette players. Hell, most of them couldn't read the print catalogs they had been sent or manipulate the controls on the cassette players they had received. What sense did it make for a "library for the blind and physically handicapped" to send out print catalogs, why not send out catalogs on tape or disc?

This is part of the reason I went back to school in pursuit of a Master's degree, so I could work with folks less capable than I was and who could, I felt, benefit from my knowledge. So, in August 1978 I returned to Western Michigan University for yet another year's study and graduated with a Master of Arts degree in Rehabilitation Teaching, in order to be able to work with individuals who had sustained a significant loss of vision. I wanted to teach them how to continue to be productive members of society and give them the knowledge they would need in order to be able to function with severely limited vision.

While I was in graduate school, I had the opportunity to work with a Mobility Instructor's teacher, that is, he taught Mobility Instructors how to teach a person who is blind how to get around using a cane. One of the things he taught me was how important it was for me to memorize a route, how important it was for me to be able to _l__i__s_ _t__e__n_ to what was going on around me and to be able to use my other senses; sound cues and my sense of smell to assist me in finding my way around a college campus large enough to provide schooling for more than 20,000 students. This was probably one of the most significant pieces of information I ever learned. I might have known this, here-to-fore, but it took someone's bringing it to my attention in order for it to begin to happen on a regular basis. After graduating with my Master's degree in the summer of 1979 it was on to Indiana that fall to my first job as a Rehabilitation Teacher.

After working as a teacher for several years, one afternoon a gentleman came in and gave a demonstration of talking computers. This was in the mid 80's, and up to this point, blind folks had been pretty much left out of the on-rushing computer world. There were Braille terminals available if you wanted to shell out more than $6,000.00, but it soon became apparent that with a computer with speech output and a large print magnifier, visually impaired, sighted and blind users could make use of the same files, but with different access points. This would mean that files and necessary forms to be filled out would be accessible to both sighted and blind employees alike, thus to a certain extent leveling the playing field in the work place.

Soon after this demonstration I decided to go to work for the company selling talking computers and learned much about sales, people and Braille translation software. I was involved in setting up rules for one of the first pieces of Braille translation software, in 1983. This was also the year that I attended a consumer convention in Philadelphia and with the blessing of my boss we purchased 6,000 catalogs in Braille to be given out at consumer conventions that year. We were one of the first companies to do this for blind consumers. I'm not sure how many sales we accrued out of that effort, but we certainly were well-received by anyone who read Braille at the conventions.

In 1985 I moved on into telemarketing for a while and in 1988 I tried my hand at my own business. Then I moved to Charleston, South Carolina where I learned to cope with hurricanes and worked at a resource center for blind adults. After that I moved back to Michigan where I became a parent and then on to Ohio and now Missouri. I've been very lucky, I've been able to go where I've wanted to go, whenever I've felt I needed to go. And now, it's on to another endeavor into the internet and what it has to offer. In some cases, I've had to have a talk with myself about moving. It's not easy for someone who is blind to move. There are things like public transportation, jobs and where to live and let's not forget about the need for accessible areas via sidewalks and intersections which are fairly easily crossed without multiple streets coming together and this is just the beginning.

When I was doing my internship for my Master's degree, my supervising instructor was Bob Utrup. Bob had written a book about the necessary information a person who is blind needs in order to be able to select an apartment. Could that be my next book, to revise his work with some added information for everyone, not just people who are blind?

I hope after reading this book that you will find out that although you or someone you know may have suffered a significant loss of vision that you or they can continue to function with some assistance from family members and friends, or with training, regain the necessary skills to go on with your life.

Yes, there are lots of things to think about if one loses a significant amount of vision or becomes completely blind. After reading this book you will have a better understanding of what those items are, and how blind and visually impaired people learn to cope and do, daily. Just because you, or someone in your family has sustained a significant loss of vision doesn't mean you or they can't continue to contribute. Through the rehabilitation process and by developing a network of friends and support systems through organizations like the NFB and ACB and the Blinded Veterans of America and by learning to make use of your other senses you can learn to deal with vision loss, and very well.

FAMILY MEMBERS AND VISION LOSS

Understanding, supporting and participating

Dealing With Vision Loss

ADJUSTING TO VISION LOSS

If you are a family member of someone who is experiencing vision loss, it's probably not much fun for either you or them. There are a number of things which you need to understand, and maybe if you do, it will make things much easier for you and the person experiencing the trauma of vision loss.

First of all, they are scared. Their life is being turned upside down. They are, to a certain degree, losing their independence, their financial security, and their sense of self-worth because they don't have the same abilities as they did when they had normal vision.

Vision loss is not at all an easy thing to deal with. In fact, studies have shown vision loss is one of the most feared losses which can occur to an individual.

Certainly, if you look at vision loss from your standpoint, that is, an individual with normal vision, you would be nearly terrified if you lost your vision tomorrow. Think about it, you wouldn't know how to function. You would lose your personal independence in that you would not be able for the most part to get around on your own, at least for a while, safely. You would no longer blend into the community because if you had suffered a severe enough loss of vision so as not to be able to determine whether a light at an intersection was red or green you would need to use a cane so that drivers and other pedestrians would know you had sustained a vision loss. Your friends and family would believe that they couldn't count on you any

Fred Olver

more because of their own fears about vision loss. Not because you were or are any less capable, but because their perception of you and your abilities would be colored by their own perceptions of what it would be like for them if they suffered a severe loss of vision. As a result of all of this, your self-esteem is bound to be affected. At times you feel that no one believes in you any more, in fact, it's hard for you to believe in yourself, because you feel so inadequate. The result of this is that one's entire personality under-goes a rebirth. It is said that in a sense the person who could see and had normal vision dies and the person who is now legally blind is born. At this point total re-organization of a person's psyche takes place, that is, learning to live being blind[1].

There are differences in the perception of the impact of vision loss on a individual. One consumer organization goes so far as to say that vision loss can be reduced to a mere inconvenience. That may be true for individuals who look at it from the standpoint of having grown up with vision loss from birth, however for those people who experience extreme vision loss beyond the age of twenty-one, losing one's vision or a large portion of it can and will be, for a while extremely difficult to deal with.

With the onset of vision loss or blindness, whether legal or total, one does, whether he/she wants to admit it or not, lose a certain amount of financial and occupational independence. Employers aren't always willing to keep an employee after they have suffered a substantial vision

---

[1] *Blindness: What it is, What it does, and How to live with it,* By Father Thomas J. Carroll Published by Little, Brown and Company, Boston, MA.

Dealing With Vision Loss

loss. I have known individuals, who, after losing most of their vision been asked to retire early. True, without the necessary skills in order to continue in a job, an individual probably needs to consider this as an option, or, if nothing else, take a leave of absence in order to acquire new skills or to determine whether or not they want to continue in the job at all. And what happens if they leave their job? Well, then they have to live off there savings, if they have any, or ask for the help of other family members, and apply for Social Security benefits just as soon as possible.

Okay, so you've got this relative or friend, and they've lost most of their vision, so what now? They may not be able to appreciate a football game any more from the stands, so they may now want to listen to it on the radio or watch the game on TV. They may not be able to enjoy it in the same way, but they can still enjoy it in a different way. A person may not be able to enjoy an exhibit at the museum in the same way they did before their loss of vision. But many museums offer taped information to patrons who need it in order to enjoy the exhibitions and so they need not skip the trip. Just because a person has limited vision doesn't mean they can't do something, they may just choose to do it differently.

This seems like a good time to bring to your attention the fact that you gain as much as 90% of your information through your vision. It now becomes necessary for the person who is going through the process of adjusting to vision loss to learn how to compensate for this loss by learning to gain the same information using their other senses. One of the suggestions I would make to my students was to watch the

Fred Olver

TV show "MASH." The reason I did so was because so much of what goes on is done with sound cues so that a person doesn't have to keep their eyes glued to the screen in order to follow what is going on.

Another way to continue to watch TV together is to keep in mind that oftentimes networks such as TNT and TBS have (SAP) Secondary Audio Programming available for use with some of their programs. This can be activated through the menus on your television or VHS recorder. Turner Classic Movies channel also lists in their schedule which movies have (DVS) Descriptive Video Services available for blind and visually impaired users and some networks like TBS, TNT and USA network list on their web sites which programs have SAP available for their viewers.

Most libraries for the blind and even some public libraries have descriptive videos available. I have been collecting movies now for more than four years and have a collection of over twenty-five hundred movies, including two silent movies, and none of them with descriptive video. Granted, most of the movies I have in my collection are older, and that is because older movies tend to have more dialog than the newer movies. Remember, I learned to watch TV without actually seeing it, kind of like having a radio with a glass window in the front of it.

The World of Communications

In a sense we've talked about communications when we speak about watching TV, however if you think about

Dealing With Vision Loss

it there is much more to communications than that. Communications is writing a check for your credit card payment, it is reading the telephone bill and looking at the advertisements which come in the mail each week. Without communications, or the ability to communicate, an individual is in deep trouble. So, how do we compensate for this deficit in communications?

In most communities there is access to what are called radio reading services or radio information services. Most generally these services can be found out about through libraries for the blind. They offer programming, sometimes 24 hours a day, reading area newspapers, grocery ads, books and magazines.

A second source of excellent information is ACB Radio available on the internet at http://www.acbradio.org. Besides offering old-time radio and a café where only music put together or written by blind musicians is performed, they also offer another stream of informational programs presented by blind individuals on such things as cooking, adjustment to vision loss, doing things around the house and various aspects of technology. The last stream of information available for non-English speaking individuals is now available on their site as well. Go to their web site to find out more information about these offerings.

A third means of gaining information is NFB NEWSLINE®, [2] a nationwide telephone service provided by the National

---

[2] NFB-NEWSLINE® is a registered trademark of the National Federation of the Blind.

Fred Olver

Federation of the Blind. NEWSLINE® offers local newspapers, magazines and much, much more.

Okay, so now your brother or sister or mom is back in the loop in getting information but what about paying those bills? I myself have opted to have funds paid out of my checking account each month. I receive the bill as I had in the past, and on the due date the money is withdrawn from my account. Check with your utilities and bank to see if statements can be made available in large print or if the information can be accessed over the phone. If one is not comfortable with automatic withdrawal, one can always punch in their ATM card number in order to perform each monthly transaction over the telephone. Also, some banks will provide individuals with large print checks, and even some offer checks with raised lines so a person can determine where the necessary information is to be placed by touch on the check. In the case of individuals wanting information in Braille, some utilities will send out statements in this format as well. Can you imagine living until you are 54 and not having had access to your bank statements, phone and utility bills in a readable format?

Another part of this communications thing is being able to meet with and get to know other people who are experiencing similar challenges. There are three organizations of blind folks in the United States, the NFB, the ACB and the BVA. The first two organizations have affiliates in most states, divisions and special interest groups dealing with most types of activities whether they are related to work home or recreational activities and everything in between. It needs to be pointed out that

Dealing With Vision Loss

both the NFB and ACB have organizations for parents of blind children and these organizations are excellent resources for children and parents alike. Oftentimes senior citizen's centers may have support groups for individuals having sustained a vision loss and parents can look to other school districts in their area to find other parents who have children with similar difficulties.

In The Home

When a person loses some or most of their vision, they're probably not going to want to go many places until they become more comfortable functioning with their vision loss. It may take several times of asking for them to want to go out to eat, go shopping, or out to a senior center. Consequently, the home is the place where they want and need to feel safe, first, and then to extend that safety net for themselves outside the home. This is where Rehabilitation Teachers and Orientation and Mobility instructors become necessary. As pointed out elsewhere these individuals and the training they provide are most necessary in order for your friend or family member to maintain sufficient skills which will allow them to continue to function as a participant in the community.

This process begins by finding the nearest state office of services for the blind or Division of Blind Services. Here they will have to deal with an application to fill out. It's a good idea to have a recent eye report to attach to the application and information about any other health issues as well. Usually a mobility instructor, rehabilitation teacher or rehabilitation counselor sees the person first. During this

Fred Olver

interview information about possible training programs is given, much paperwork is completed, release forms are signed and the individual conducting the interview tries to get a general idea of what the individuals' needs are. Sometimes a second appointment is set up during which a low vision evaluation is completed: and an evaluation of an individual's daily living skills or Orientation and Mobility evaluation is begun.

During these evaluations, skills like getting around the home or neighborhood, telling time, and cooking skills are evaluated. In short, anything that an individual might need to do around his/her home is fair game, especially for the rehabilitation teacher since they teach most of the skills which a person may need to re-learn in order to maintain his/her independence. Oftentimes this re-learning is nothing more than pointing out the ridges on the rim of a quarter or dime, how to separate paper money, or where to purchase a talking watch or Braille timer or marking one's stove at various temperatures with glue or nail polish so as to make a raised bump or two to line up, one on the dial, and one on the stove so that when the dots line up the temperature would be set for 350° or 425°F.

With regard to other skills like learning Braille, or use of the abacus, acquiring these skills can take as long as six to eight months, and for folks learning new job skills, leaving home to attend a training center for specific training may be the only means of acquiring necessary skills to gain employment. If it is possible for one to attend a rehabilitation center, this is most definitely the better choice because skill areas are presented on a more consistent

Dealing With Vision Loss

basis, and the experience of attending a rehabilitation center can prove to be invaluable from the stand-point of meeting and getting to know other people who are going through the same kinds of problems and difficulties. This is not to say that needed skills such as Braille or use of the abacus in order to keep track of one's check book or put phone numbers on for a short period of time until they can be transferred to a tape recorder or in to Braille can not be learned while at home, the process just takes longer, because oftentimes the Rehabilitation Teacher may only be able to see students once a month. An alternative might be to take a course, such as Braille or abacus, through the Hadley School. They offer courses in a myriad of areas and subjects and if desired, one can get one's GED.

ACCEPTANCE OF VISION LOSS

When your mom sister aunt or dad has done all of these things they're probably well on their way to re-asserting themselves in to society. This isn't going to happen overnight in fact, depending on the amount of vision lost and how quickly that loss takes place can make all the difference in how one reacts to what's going on. If the onset is gradual, the trauma will be less severe. This is not to say that an individual will not experience mourning and depression, it's just that these symptoms may take longer to manifest themselves. The person who experiences a substantial vision loss is, in a sense, starting over. They are having to re-learn the same skills they learned as a child, but by using other senses, not necessarily their vision. This is not to say that an individual should not use their vision to assist, just that the use of vision may hinder them because

Fred Olver

they are trying so much harder to see when it might prove easier to listen to a book being read, or a TV show, or determining doneness of French toast by touching it with a spatula rather than looking at it.

I have been blind all of my life. I was born two months premature and was given too much oxygen while in the incubator. As a result, my eyes did not fully develop and I learned to do absolutely everything without the use of vision. I still get angry. I get frustrated at all the drivers who go by on rainy days when I'm standing at bus stops getting soaked, or waiting in the cold when it is about ten above zero. I don't always think its fair, and it probably isn't, but it causes me to appreciate it when I do get a ride to the store. But you see, I don't absolutely need that ride to the store. I don't need to rely on other people to get me places, because I have the FREEDOM to go anywhere any time I want to, using my other senses, making use of public transportation. I don't know anyone who is happy to be blind. I don't know anyone who would tell you that they have totally accepted blindness because I believe there are times when we all get frustrated with the fact that we can't do the things we might like to be able to, because we can't see well enough to drive or read manuals or find things in the store, but we manage. We make it happen. We are independent, we manage our own affairs, we participate on bowling leagues community organizations and walk-a-thons. We march on Washington, protest indiscretions of universities, fight cases in court and administer the law. Some of us make money playing music and others of us work on cars or build cabinets. I have friends who are customer service representatives, friends who baby sit,

Dealing With Vision Loss

friends who have made $100,000 a year selling food and snacks, and friends who because of other difficulties do not work. I know teachers, counselors, ham radio operators, lawyers, judges and even a lady who puts together flower baskets, and all of them are blind. People who are blind can do the same things that people who can see can, we may just do it differently, but the desire and outcome is the same, we like and want to contribute, we want to be a part of our community and we get great satisfaction from being able to do so just like you.

DEALING WITH A BLIND PERSON FOR THE FIRST TIME

The following are suggestions to keep in mind when dealing for the first time with a person who is blind. We are not super-human. We would like to be thought of as being just like you with the exception that we have a significant vision loss. We are not helpless, but we may not be able to do everything you do in the same way. Our limitations may be more evident, but we all have limitations, don't we?

1. I am not deaf. It is not necessary to raise your voice when speaking to me.

2. If we are in a restaurant together and the waiter or waitress asks you a question about me, or what I want, please tell them to speak to me. A response such as "I don't know, why not ask him?" would be in order.

Fred Olver

3. Do not assume I can not do something simply because I am blind. If you want to know you can always ask.

4. Do not pay any attention to my dog guide. Do not talk to him/her. My dog may be lovely, wag its tail, look directly at you, however it is working. When it is in harness, it is working. If you feel you must pet my dog guide, please ask if it is okay first, and if I say no, please respect my wishes. If you talk to my dog, you are distracting it from its job.

5. Blindness does not automatically ensure that my other senses will be improved. Any sensory development on my part took lots of time and awareness to develop. It doesn't happen because I can't see, I have taught myself to rely on my other senses instead of my vision.

6. I probably will not want to touch your face to determine what you look like, but feel free to tell me if there's something on the floor that needs to be cleaned up, or my shirt's a mess and needs to be changed.

7. Do not avoid the words watch or see; I use them all the time.

8. Yes, I do watch TV and I do go to movies. If we go to a movie do not feel compelled to tell me what is going on. If I need to know, I will ask you.

9. Just because I may be blind doesn't mean I can't afford to buy my meal at the restaurant.

Dealing With Vision Loss

10. Do not feed my dog, it is fed daily and does not need table scraps.

11. If my dog is doing something it ought not to be doing, please let me know so I can discipline it myself.

12. If you see someone petting my dog, please let me know so I can inform them as to whether or not it is okay for them to do so.

13. There is no such thing as a dumb question except the one you don't ask.

14. I may be glad to give you some information about being blind, however if you take the time to get to know me, you will find that I have many interests, hobbies and other activities which I pursue.

15. Because I have not ever been able to see, I do not see pictures of anything at any time, not even when I dream. However if I had been able to see at one time, I would retain those visual memories, and although they might at some point become out-of-date, they would be invaluable to me because having been able to see, I would retain the ability to visualize.

16. Blindness is not contagious. In most cases it is not hereditary and is not passed down through the generations.

17. Every single person who is blind is different. Each blind person you will meet probably has a different type

Fred Olver

of vision loss and probably sees things differently. Some are more capable than others. Some will be able to travel independently and some will ask for assistance. We do not all learn to play musical instruments at an early age and some of us can only play the radio. Please treat us with the respect we deserve and be sure to treat us as the individuals we are.

If you're sharing your life with a person who is blind you're in for a world of discoveries and growth. You'll learn that "treat me like everyone else" means that "yes, I'll need some adaptations but don't do one more thing for me than what I absolutely need." You'll learn to be more descriptive in your language; you won't say "over there" you'll say "on the dresser" or "six inches to your left" and you'll learn to do it in a way that is casual and natural and no big deal. You should keep your expectations high; because people who are blind can cook and make your coffee and take good care of you, too. You'll learn to describe anything and everything you notice that is interesting or unusual or helpful. You'll find ways to show all the beauty that you encounter through touch or sound or smell. On the other hand you could well be treated to a unique perspective: the difference between a mother and baby robin's call, the first cricket of the season, or a dove just taking off. You'll learn to pay close attention to the wonders of all your senses. You'll learn that being fully human doesn't depend upon the possession of sight. Expect to enjoy the learning process because it can go on forever.

Dealing With Vision Loss

THE REALITY OF BLINDNESS

Let's take a closer look at some of the statistics available on blindness and visual impairment. I think you'll be rather surprised. First of all understand that there is some disparity in these statistics. The reasons for this are:

1. It has been quite some time since these statistics were compiled.
2. There is no exact way to be able to measure or to gain a solid numbers of blind people in this country because short of asking all blind folks to register it just can't be done.
3. Each agency compiling statistics uses a different measure in determining their numbers. That is to say that depending on which statistic you read, the definition of individuals perceived to be in a particular group may be different. In some cases there is only one statistic available so that statistic must stand on its own.

It is an accepted fact that the unemployment or under-employment rate of people who are considered blind is right around 70%. This means that only 30% of those blind folks who have an education, comparable to their sighted counter-parts, are employed. This is so "not" acceptable. If any other segment of the population of this country was thought to be in this circumstance they would be bringing down the walls of Jericho. Even if you take in to account the fact that it is suggested that 35% of those who are considered to be blind are over the age of 65 and the fact that only half of those individuals between the ages of 22

17

Fred Olver

and 50 are employed, the employment rate among people who are blind falls far short of what it should be.

Let's take a look at the use of Braille. According to the National Federation of the Blind, on their web site excluding deaf-blind children, as updated in 2002, there are some 82,000 legally blind children in the United States. According to the American Printing House for the Blind only some 5,500 children in the United States were making use of Braille as of 1995. At the time this statistic was made available that figure represented only 10% of those children who were considered legally blind. One reason for this is that several states do not require their teachers of blind children to have knowledge of Braille. A supposed argument against the use of Braille is the ability to be able to make use of talking computers. That is to say that use of computers is oftentimes given as a reason not to have to teach the student who might be able to use Braille in tandem with computers. What results at the time of graduation is that these children who have not learned Braille are considered to be functionally illiterate because they have no means of writing or reading except with computer or tape player. This also means that they would not be able to learn to play cards, Monopoly, Scrabble, read elevators or room doors in hotels, or signs outside restroom doors, and let's not forget the book titles of the tapes and other recordings they may receive from their library for the blind. They would have no access to a number of magazines which are only available in Braille from the Library of Congress and all of the books which are made available in Braille. What happens in the future when the Library of Congress asks for funding to produce

Dealing With Vision Loss

Braille books and only 5% of all those people who are blind are said to be able to read Braille? To be fair, there is one caveat to the statistic on Braille. There is no measure of those children who are considered multi-handicapped and for whatever reason can not, have not or would not be able to learn to use Braille. I believe this may be off-set though by the numbers of deaf-blind children and their possible use of Braille as a method of communication. But even if you add another 10,000 to the number making that number some 93,000 the numbers of children using Braille is appallingly low.

In 1990 it was reported that only 109,000 individuals made use of long canes. In today's numbers this means that less than 10% of those considered to be legally blind would have learned to use a cane then 90% of blind individuals are traveling around unsafely, at risk, in danger of being killed because they have not been told that they need to make use of a cane. That 109,000 represents less than 10% of the number of individuals who were thought to be legally blind as of 1994-95 as mentioned on the web site of the American Foundation for the Blind.

Yet another piece of this pie and perhaps the most important piece of information is the fact that there is absolutely no agreement with regard to the numbers of blind people in the United States. According to The American Foundation for the Blind in 1994 there were 1.3 million blind folks in the United States, with one person losing their vision every seven minutes. If you take this out to the year 2007 that would have added some 846,000 individuals to that group. Prevent Blindness America says, according

Fred Olver

to the 2000 census there are 119,000,000 individuals in the baby boomer generation who are at risk of becoming blind. If only 10% of this group develop severe vision loss that would mean that some twelve million people would experience severe vision loss over the next 20-30 years. The NFB says, that according to a study done in 1990 carried out through the next 10 to 25 years that only 1.6 million people in 2015 and by the year 2030 some 2.4 million people will be affected.

If you take any one of these statistics and you look at it closely enough, I believe you will find that the best interests of people who are blind are not being served. The unemployment/under-employment rate, the use of canes among blind folks, the teaching of Braille to children and, as described elsewhere in this book rehabilitation programs for adults all fall short in meeting the needs of blind folks in the United States.

I am well-acquainted with one state agency which recently had an opening for a Rehabilitation Teacher. One of the requirements was that each of the candidates for the position had to take and pass a Braille Proficiency test. None of the candidates for the job passed the test, the job was not re-posted and one of the candidates who had previously applied for the job was hired in spite of the fact that she was unable to make use of, and consequently teach Braille to her students. This agency is one which does not require Rehabilitation Teachers to be trained in the field of Rehabilitation in order to gain employment as a Rehabilitation Teacher, in fact in their job description and requirements there is no mention of Rehabilitation

Dealing With Vision Loss

teaching. I believe firmly that the quality of the outcome of rehabilitation is directly related to the quality of the instructors doing the training. If you have quality instructors the caliber of the finished product will be higher than if you do not. The same would undoubtedly be true of the teachers school districts hire to work with their blind and visually impaired children.

AN INTRODUCTION TO BLINDNESS

Several years ago, I was asked to speak to a group of students at a university near Detroit. When the instructor picked me up she proceeded to give me an outline of the topics she wanted me to cover. As I looked at the list, I noticed there were about 20 items, and I felt it would be rather difficult to cover each of them adequately. When I arrived at the university and was introduced to the class, I started speaking. Two and a half hours later, I was finished. My throat hurt from talking so long but I felt a certain amount of excitement. One of the reasons I am writing this book is because I feel I have so much to offer, in terms of experience, having been blind all of my life and knowledge, not only from the books I have read, as a result of my years of experience as a Rehabilitation Teacher but through as well my day-to-day activities and interaction with both sighted and blind individuals. The excitement I felt speaking to that group of college students is still there for me today. I doubt if it will ever go away when the prospect of speaking to a group of individuals presents itself, or taking the opportunity to educate an individual or group as to the abilities of people who are blind. I do not have the notes from that speech, but used it

Fred Olver

as a spring-board to giving a speech three or four years ago at a university in Ohio. Here is that speech.

As I stand here before you this afternoon, what was the first thing that went through your mind when you saw me? Was it that I am going to stand up here and give a lecture? Was it that you can hardly wait to hear what I have to say? As I stand here, before you, I expect the first thing you thought about was the fact that I am blind. The question then is, did you look at me as being blind first and then a person, or was the reverse true? I rather expect the former would be the case. Now, let's take a look at your perception of blindness. What were your thoughts concerning me, and my coping skills with blindness. Did you decide that if you were blind that it would be most difficult for you to cope with a loss of vision, and did you wonder how I manage to cope with it?

Most likely the answer to these questions is again yes. Ah, but you see, your perception of blindness is based, not on my terms of dealing with it, but on the basis of your having been able to see, while my point of reference is just the opposite, as I have never been able to see. So, how does one cope with blindness? Simply put, it depends on their point of reference whether that is, having been blind since birth, or as an individual having lost their vision as an adult.

In the case of children having been born blind or losing their vision very early in life, their development may not be as rapid as a sighted child, simply because children who are blind are often not exposed to the same stimuli as

Dealing With Vision Loss

children with sight. If however, taught the necessary skills to function with little or no vision, children who have been blind from a very early age can keep up with their sighted peers. These skills may include dressing one's self, use of Braille, or low vision aids in the case of children who have some usable vision, orientation and mobility and use of computers. For adults who lose their sight as a result of accident or disease, it may be necessary that they re-learn some of the skills they acquired as a child using their remaining senses in order to function at the same level they did before they lost their vision. These skills might include: Braille, adaptive cooking skills, orientation and mobility; use of a white cane, and in the case of most people desiring to further their education, some type of computer skills training.

Let's say you are, for the first time, confronted with the situation of having to meet with, or deal with someone who is blind, what do you do? Should you avoid the words blind, or see, do you use the word sightless, so as not to hurt the person's feelings? What if you are asked to show them where the bathroom is, do you go in with them? And how do you get them there in the first place?

Should you avoid the words blind or see? I doubt it. I know I'm blind, you know I'm blind, so there it is. I find myself watching TV, just like the rest of you. Blindness only refers to my eyes not my ability to discern what is going on around me, or to understand spoken or written word. True, I may have to do things a bit different from you, and I may not go see Marcel Marceau the next time he is in town, but in most situations, people who are blind

Fred Olver

can do just fine if they are taught how to orient themselves to where they are in relation to the area they are in and learn to discern what is going on around them by making use of environmental cues.

Each state has an agency to provide services to blind and visually impaired individuals. In most cases these services are separate from those available to the usual candidate for services of the vocational rehabilitation agency. There are libraries which offer books on cassette and in large print, and oftentimes radio reading services which provide free receivers to individuals with limited vision from which one can hear community newspapers being read, magazines not available in alternative formats, and books which might not otherwise be available to the person who is blind.

The NFB, the largest of three consumer organizations of people who are blind boasts a membership of 50,000 people; and is the organization most often responsible for sponsoring legislation concerning the needs of people who are blind. Besides being responsible for Braille Literacy laws in more than half of the states, the Federation offers a monthly magazine, The Braille Monitor. The NFB holds a convention each year the first week of July which provides information about technology, as well as constructive debates with organizations that feel it is necessary to be caretakers of the blind. The Federation also offers training at facilities, one each, in Colorado, Minnesota and Louisiana. Through Louisiana Tech University one can take advanced degree training in the areas of Orientation and Mobility and teacher training programs for individuals who want

Dealing With Vision Loss

to be involved in the blind rehabilitation process as role models which promulgate the NFB philosophy. Besides consumer organizations there are companies like Maxi-Aids and Independent Living Aids, which sell Braille and large print watches, canes, computer games and a myriad of other aids for blind and visually impaired people. Once an individual is considered to be legally blind, they will become eligible for benefits through the Social Security Administration. Depending how much they have or have not worked, they may be eligible for benefits based on what they earned, and how long they earned it.

So, you're in your office, someone gives you a note, all you see is a name. You go out front to get the person, and oh gees, they're blind. What do you do? Being a guide for someone who is blind is comparatively easy. Most of us know how to be guided, some may refuse; however if you'll just ask the person if they would like to take your arm they will probably do so, and off you go. In the case of those people making use of a dog-guide, do not talk to the dog, it is working. Do not reach down to pet the dog, and do not offer to get the dog a cookie. It is working.

Position yourself most often to the left of the person and ask them if they'd like to take your arm. When they do, it should be just above the elbow. When you go through a doorway, which may be narrower, take your hand and place it behind your back, just above your hips. This will inform the person who is blind that they need to drop their hand down to your wrist and straighten their arm so as to be following directly behind you through the narrower doorway. Once you get through the doorway, bring your

25

Fred Olver

arm back to your side and the person following should move their hand up again to just above the elbow. Once you get to your office, explain to the person where you want them to sit. They should be able to find the chair with their cane, however if they don't have a cane with them, try to position them in front of the chair and let them know where they are in relation to it. When the interview is over with, and you want the person to sign something, just ask them how they would like you to line them up in order to put their signature in the right place.

With regard to those folks who have dogs, they will most likely have the dog follow you to your office. It is a good idea to let them know when you are going to turn, and which way you are turning. Speak to the person, (not the dog.) Again, once you get to the office, let them know where the chair is you want them to sit in, and the dog should help the person find the chair.

In closing, let me say this to you. After I had decided to get an earring about five years ago, I did some thinking as to why I had done so. I decided this. If I see a man walking down the street who is blind, I might say to myself, "hmmm there goes a man who is blind." However if I see a man walking down the street that is blind and has an earring, I might say or think to myself "now that man has something to say."

DIMINISHED VISION AND YOU

Getting around, overcoming barriers and reclaiming your life.

Dealing With Vision Loss

ENCOUNTERING DIMINISHED VISION

Blindness is a terrible thing for an individual to have to go through. It causes one to have to re-think how to do simple things like tell time, read a newspaper, dial a telephone, set the thermostat, cook and/or identify money. Depending on how severe the loss of vision, you may not even realize you have suffered a loss of vision until you go outside at night, or have a traffic accident. Vision loss can occur to anyone of any age, however those most often affected are senior citizens. There are three main causes of vision loss among this group. These are: diabetes, macular degeneration and glaucoma. This is not to say that there are not other causes of vision loss, only that these are the ones which occur most often. So it becomes more important for older individuals to have their vision checked more frequently, especially those in whose families these problems have already occurred. Have it checked at least once a year if not every six months. Whether an individual has any of these three dysfunctions in their vision, in most cases, the difficulties with vision will come on slowly. Thus the effects of vision loss may go unnoticed for a long period of time before they would be considered significant. However if you have not noticed any problems with your vision and all of a sudden you do, again, you need to seek immediate attention from your physician or ophthalmologist.

It is a fact that for most people over the age of forty vision changes will occur. Oftentimes these changes require one to think about using bifocals, but for about 10% extreme vision loss will take place. In some cases this loss of vision will be very slow to happen and for others the loss of vision

Fred Olver

will take place in a relatively short period of time. The most prevalent cause of vision loss is macular degeneration. Diabetes is a close second and glaucoma third. In each case vision loss can represent significant losses in abilities and can cause one to have to under-go significant learning in order to compensate for the loss of vision however none of these has to represent the end of independence.

In the case of macular degeneration, you may experience loss of vision in the center of your visual field, that is to say that you may find yourself looking at things more from the side rather than straight on, and indeed, this problem may not be the same in both eyes. It is sometimes referred to as a blind spot in the center of one's vision. It will cause you problems when trying to read, looking at items straight in front of you and even seeing people's faces will at some point become more difficult.

In the case of diabetes, you may be seeing floaters in your vision, or be having blind spots in your vision. These floaters or blind spots can be caused by blood vessels in the back of the eye weakening and breaking open causing blood flow and scar tissue to form. They may also be caused by laser treatments designed to stem the growth of unwanted blood vessels in the back of the eye. These blind spots do not usually occur for a long period of time after one has become diabetic. Again, if one notices either of these symptoms, they need to contact their physician or ophthalmologist as soon as possible.

With regard to glaucoma, there are several types, however the most significant symptoms are that you may be seeing

Dealing With Vision Loss

halos around lights and/or you may be experiencing extremely bad headaches.

We've talked just a bit about the signs related to vision loss with each of these three problems, but lets get beyond that and talk about specific limitations. Please understand these are all maybes, they all don't necessarily have to occur at the same time but they all are signs that definite vision loss has taken place

Difficulty Driving

This is probably the most significant problem, or the one which would be recognized first. Maybe you can't see the signs as well as you used to, or read addresses as well. Maybe you have difficulty telling when it's okay to change lanes or seeing the traffic. In any case, if you're having difficulty driving, you need to have someone drive you to a doctor's appointment to find out just how bad your vision is. One friend of mine found he had significant vision loss when he drove in to a bridge abutment at 50 miles per hour. He wasn't injured badly, but he did at that point have to acknowledge the fact that he was no longer able to drive. No one likes to admit they can't do something whether it is because of getting older, or vision loss or limited range of motion. I didn't like giving up playing beep baseball, but the fact is that I just don't have the agility any more and can't get down on the ground nearly as fast as I used to.

Fred Olver

Difficulty Reading

Another significant problem which can occur is that it becomes much more difficult to read. You've probably been to the drug store to sample their short list of magnifiers, and if you're lucky, maybe you've borrowed one or two magnifiers from a friend or a family member has purchased one for you. But after a while, the magnifiers don't help any more. It becomes more and more frustrating for you to read and write out your bills. You purchase a new address book so you can write your addresses out in larger print and you purchase hi-lighters to assist you in being able to see what you have written. And you are wondering, what do I do next? What do I do if my vision gets worse? I like my home and want to stay in it, I don't want to be a burden to any of my children, but I don't want to move in to a nursing home!

So, What's Next?

Let's talk about feelings. How are you going to feel? Well, mostly scared. How are you going to get places, what if you lose all of your vision, what's going to happen next? Nobody has the answers to all of these questions for you. You may lose more vision, but chances are you'll always have some of it. Yes, it's going to change your life, but with a good attitude, the changes don't have to make that much difference. There's going to be a period of adjustment while you get used to the idea that you are visually impaired or even legally blind, but with the right training and understanding you can still continue to function pretty much as you did with normal vision.

Dealing With Vision Loss

Let's try and look at the positives, but first of all, give yourself a break. Understand that probably for quite sometime you aren't going to want to do anything. Go with it. Accept it, don't let it bring you down any further than you can handle. Maybe individual counseling is a possibility, or counseling for you and your spouse, and maybe even the kids, too. You may not be able to drive any more, but it doesn't mean it's the end of the world. Try to find resources within your community like public transportation (door-to-door) services which you can make use of in order to get to doctor's appointments or shopping. These services will pick you up at home and drop you off at the doctor's office or store and return to pick you up later. Other resources may include senior citizen's centers or maybe there is a support group for people who are experiencing vision loss which meets at the local library. Also, you need to get in touch with your state rehabilitation agency so that a determination can be made as to whether you are eligible for their services. Depending on such factors as age, income, and amount of vision loss you may find that you are eligible for all kinds of services including training, visual aids and/or possible restoration. If your vision loss is severe enough your local library can steer you in the direction of area libraries for the blind. If you have had a significant vision loss and you feel you would benefit from contact with others who are visually impaired or legally blind you might also want to contact the NFB, BVA or the ACB. The ACB and NFB have affiliates in each state and you may find that there is a local chapter in your area.

Okay, so you've found out your vision is getting worse. You have noticed that you're having difficulty reading the

Fred Olver

newspaper, setting your stove, or identifying money and telling time, what do you do?

The answers to these questions are not easy, or short. In fact, adjusting to vision loss can turn out to be fairly difficult, at best. The first thing I would suggest you do is to get in touch with your physician or ophthalmologist to determine just how much your vision has decreased. By doing that, you will begin to be able to map out a strategy for dealing with vision loss. The second thing I would suggest as mentioned above is that you find out whether or not there is a chapter of either the NFB or ACB in your immediate area and try to get in touch with one of their members. By doing so, you will immediately be in contact with other people like yourself who have a vision problem, and you'll find that most of them are more than willing to help with any questions you might have or just to be there for you to talk to if you need someone to listen. If there's not a chapter in your area, then, surely there is a state affiliate of both of these organizations, and if you're a veteran you might also want to get hold of the Blinded Veterans of America.

Don't worry if you don't want to get hold of anyone for the moment. Don't feel bad if you're scared to death of what may be happening to you, or what your doctor has told you about your vision loss. Perhaps the one bright spot is that there's a good chance that you will not lose all of your vision, which means that you'll probably have a small portion of your vision to rely on, this isn't always true, but generally speaking, some 80% to 90% of all people who are considered legally blind maintain some usable vision.

Dealing With Vision Loss

LIVING INDEPENDENTLY IN THE 21ST CENTURY

The process of rehabilitation can be a long and arduous task with many obstacles to overcome and steps to be taken which will allow you to get back to the same point you were at before you became aware of the fact that you had suffered a substantial loss of vision. It began when you were confronted with the fact that you were no longer able to drive, or had to find new and different means of accomplishing the tasks which you had previously completed while using your vision to its fullest extent.

According to the Academy for Certification of Vision Rehabilitation and Education Professionals (http://www. acvrep.org) the definition of rehabilitation is the re-learning of skills necessary to complete the tasks of daily living by making use of compensatory skills in exchange for ones which are limited or changed as a result of trauma, accident or changes in ability due to life circumstances. These changes, in your case vision, require you to seek other means to gain the same information, which you formerly gained through the use of your vision. Previous to this point in your life, you received up to 90% of your information visually. It is now up to you to gain that same information with your other senses. This means that instead of your other senses: smell, touch, hearing and taste being auxiliary senses, you now have to learn to use them as primary senses in order to substitute for vision loss. In order to accomplish this task you must go through a re-learning process, finding different ways to accomplish the same goals, which you may have taken for granted in the past.

Fred Olver

Walking to the store may seem an awesome task at this time, however with diligence and work walking to the store will again be within your grasp. True, you may not be able to do it visually, however by learning to use a cane and using both hearing and touch you can gain similar information as you might have formerly gained with your vision, thus allowing you to complete this task successfully. As has been mentioned elsewhere in this book, there are several components involved in the rehabilitation process.

- A desire to go on with your life being visually limited
- Receiving training in areas relating to daily living skills, if necessary
- Setting goals for yourself
  and
- Convincing yourself that you can do and learning to do most of the same things you did using your remaining vision along with your other senses.

As part of the rehabilitation process there are several areas which are necessary for one to delve into in order that one might be able to continue to care for one's self. These include basic skills in the following areas:

- Braille
- Mobility
- Abacus
- Computer skills
- Use of low vision aids
- Cooking
- Home management

Dealing With Vision Loss

Substitutes:

For Braille: Use of a tape recorder
Mobility: makes use of volunteers and door-to-door transportation
Abacus: Has someone else handle your checkbook
Computer skills: Make use of a reader to gain information
Cooking: Eat out, if you can afford it, or find someone to always cook for you
Home Management: Live with someone else and have them do all the necessary tasks of caring for your home, or live in an apartment complex where most of your needs are taken care of, such as repairs, cutting grass, etc.

The Why's of These Skills?

Braille is often considered the best and most functional substitute for print. Although only about 15% of blind people make use of it, Braille can prove to be most functional for any of the things you may have used print for including:

- making lists
- phone numbers
- keeping track of your checkbook
- labeling CD's, cassettes or food items just to name a few.

Mobility is the key to your independence. Undoubtedly you could get around when you had more vision, so what's to stop you now. The white cane is the key to safe travel.

Fred Olver

Without it, drivers, clerks and others may not understand the reasons you do some of the things you do. If you cut someone off while walking, if you trip over a step or curb, miss a chair or not see where someone is pointing, a cane will be an immediate explanation for your difficulties. Besides being an indicator of vision loss, the cane is also an extension of your hand. It can tell you when you've reached the bottom of the steps, how deep that curb is and is the item with which you find those bicycles which miraculously seem to appear in the sidewalk when you want to go out for an evening stroll or up to the store for a gallon of milk.

The abacus is a tool, invented by the Chinese approximately 2,000 years ago for computational purposes and is still in use today. The abacus, which we use, is a modified one, so that the beads do not move as easily from top to bottom. It can be used for addition, subtraction, multiplication and division, figuring percentages and keeping track of your checkbook and telephone numbers. The abacus has 13 columns for placement of numbers, and no memory functions, so the numbers if they are to be saved need to be put either into Braille, written down, if using large print or on a cassette tape before the abacus can be used for the next chore.

The fourth area of endeavor is not for everyone. It is one which can be most useful on the job or at home. The flexibility which it allows is practically boundless. The computer, desktop, laptop, or modified computer terminal for use by blind individuals can turn out to be one of your most functional tools if used properly. As a tool for

Dealing With Vision Loss

gathering information from the www, the computer has no rival. Indeed, while putting this book together, I sat at my desk and spent several hundred hours with my word processing and screen-reading software preparing the text and making necessary changes. On a computer with large print software or screen-reading speech software, I can send and receive e-mail, have conversations with people around the world or across the street, look up movie or TV listings make my flight reservations or go shopping for my Christmas gifts.

Low vision aids are magnifiers and large print books. They allow you to continue to function visually as much as possible while learning to make use of your other senses. The trick is to determine whether it makes more sense to use magnifiers to continue to function visually or to learn Braille and try to make use of that form of communication or make use of synthetic speech in order to accomplish specific tasks. If you want to continue to use your computer you may find that software which enlarges the size of the letters on the screen in concert with speech output allows you the ability to read visually what is on the screen and back that up with the spoken word of speech output (available with Zoom-Text).

Cooking is the next area of concern, since most of us like to eat. Whether you were a chef before you lost some of your vision or just an out-of-the-can man, the kitchen can be a fun place to be. You have the choice of what you want to eat and when. If you want to, you can look up coupons on the www and thus save yourself some money. You can

Fred Olver

create your shopping list either in Braille, on tape, or using your computer, you can print it out.

The last area, home management can be a rewarding experience for the individual who has a creative mind and their own home. Whether you wish to make cabinets, re-model rooms, replace a vanity in the bathroom or just unclog a trap, this area can be a lot of fun. It's all in how you approach it. For some, though, apartments or condos where the work is done for you may prove to be more to your liking.

Besides these areas of concern, there are other questions, which you need to consider in living independently.
1. How are you going to get from your home to the store or bank?
2. Are there sidewalks in your neighborhood?
3. Can you travel safely from place to place, not putting yourself or your children in danger?
4. What are you willing to do to put yourself in the most positive living situation in order to deal with the limitations presented to you with regard to vision loss?

Now, let's look at independence. What is independence, anyway? Independence is allowing yourself the flexibility to do what you want, or can, and also allowing others to assist you when you feel it is necessary. This does not mean allowing others to do something for you because they feel you can't do it yourself, but having the guts to admit you need help. Perhaps you don't need help crossing that street; on the other hand, maybe you do need help finding something on the shelf while shopping at the store.

Dealing With Vision Loss

What can we do to enhance our independence? Independence is a wonderful word. It is a word which gives us power over ourselves and others. We say we are independent, and to some of us that means that we don't need anyone's help. We may be an independent traveler, we may be independent in the kitchen we may be an independent voter, but, sooner or later we're going to have to ask for help with something, so get used to the idea. So, maybe we aren't that independent after all, maybe we're interdependent, which to me means that I know when I need help and have the freedom and knowledge that I can ask others for help and maintain my self-esteem.

Is it right to always rely on our significant other for assistance?

The short answer is no! Just because you have lost some of your vision doesn't make you helpless. It doesn't mean you can't, it just means you need to try to learn different ways of doing things. Think about asking your spouse whether or not they mind doing that thing you think you can't do or if they will help you to learn how to do it yourself.

Books and Newspapers

I'm not going to tell you that being blind, adjusting to it, learning new ways of doing things is easy, however if one is considered legally blind they can get an extra exemption on their federal tax return. There are also discounts available with regard to mailing information to other folks who are blind and you're not alone. There are anywhere from 2.1 to five million individuals in the

Fred Olver

United States who are legally blind or visually impaired, in fact, one of them might just live around the corner from you, or perhaps they have already started a support group at the area Senior Citizen's center in your town. If you like to read, not to worry. There's probably a library which has large print books, or audio books for you to read close by. If you like reading magazines they may also be available through a radio reading service accessible with a special radio. You can find out about either one of these resources through any local library. Also, the NFB offers NEWSLINE® a program offering various newspapers and magazines both local and nationwide accessible with your telephone. If you have a computer and access to the internet, the ACB has an internet radio station http://www.acbradio.org which offers four distinctly different streams of entertainment and information. One stream offers old-time radio shows, a second offers music written, produced or performed by blind musicians, a third stream offers programming for individuals with information on everything from cooking to computers to being a handy man, all from the perspective of being blind and as well there is a fourth stream of information for non-English speaking individuals.

THE REHABILITATION PROCESS AND BEYOND

When you are ready, you might give some thought about contacting the state rehabilitation agency, or local society for the blind. Either, or both, may offer comprehensive services with regard to use of low vision aids, adjustment to blindness, other resources in your community, activities groups and if you wish to return to work: job preparedness

Dealing With Vision Loss

skills training. Oftentimes you'll find that the individuals teaching these adaptive skills are themselves blind, and at some point in their lives may have gone through the same dilemma which you find yourself in right now. Depending on your age, and health, there are two possibilities with regard to training. One is that you may decide to attend a rehabilitation center for a period of time in order to master the necessary skills which will allow you to continue to live independently with vision loss. In these centers you may find yourself in computer training classes, learning Braille, cooking, learning to make use of low vision aids and getting to know other people just like you! As time goes on, your work will get easier, and you may even find that you're not so much concentrating on the fact that you've lost your vision, but that you're learning how to adapt to it. You may learn to use a cane, so you can cross streets safely. You may learn to use magnifiers, or what are called CCTV's which will enlarge the print so you can read books again or maybe Braille.

At best, Braille is difficult, you have to acquire a more gentle sense of touch in order to be able to decipher it, but after a while, you'll be able to read that magazine or book your friends are talking about. Don't worry if you don't master Braille during your stay at the Rehab center, the Hadley School offers a course for you to continue your studies after you have returned home. Besides, who knows, you might want to correspond with some of the folks you met. True, you could do it with cassette tapes, but think how good it will feel to write your first page of Braille and send it to a friend. You might also want to play cards with your grandchildren, or learn to play cribbage. Bingo

Fred Olver

cards are also available in large print and Braille, and it's always easier to write down your shopping list than it is to memorize it. But, honestly, you may find that your memory does get better because you may find yourself memorizing telephone numbers, routes to the store or where you left your shoes.

Speaking of shoes, there are a couple things you need to keep in mind. First of all, when you buy a pair of shoes, it will take you a short while to get used to wearing them. Remember that you are now more aware of what is going on around you, this includes under-foot as well. I remember when I was working on my Master's degree and went out to get a pair of boots. I liked the boots, but after I purchased them and started walking around in them, I found that I couldn't as easily feel inclines and declines near intersections because the soles were so much thicker than what I was used to. Of course, if you're dealing with diabetes your feet are always of great concern so you may find that you need to have your feet checked more often for blisters especially after purchasing a new pair of shoes

If attending a rehabilitation center is not an option, at some point you'll probably want to have a Rehabilitation Teacher come to your home and work with you on adapting to vision loss. These teachers work with parents who are blind, senior citizens who have suffered a vision loss and individuals who although blind since birth may have sustained further vision loss, thus making it more difficult for them to continue to function because of changed visual circumstances. These teachers teach everything from

Dealing With Vision Loss

Braille to cooking, money identification, use of low vision aids, cleaning techniques for floors, counters and tables and offer tips on organizational skills, basically any skills needed in order to allow YOU to continue to function as independently as YOU want to. When you are blind, that is having suffered enough of a vision loss to be considered legally blind, sometimes referred to as visually impaired, it becomes necessary for you to become more organized. The more organized you are, the easier it will be to find things when not being able to use your vision as much as you did.

COMPUTERS AND YOU

If you look at the resources section of this book you will find that the two most listed items are places to get bibles and places to get computer software and related materials. Bibles are probably self-explanatory. Computers? Computers are or can be as important to those who have vision limitations as they are to most sighted folks.

More and more, computers are becoming the main method of communications for everyone. There are cell phones with speech output as well as email and internet capabilities. There are hand-held and portable computers available and there are laptops and desk tops available, too. With the myriad of types of computers ever growing, it's easy to understand how important they are, not only to the business man or individual working in an office, but to the individual who is at home and wants to be able to access the newspaper that you used to receive on a daily or weekly basis at your front door or email from your kids

45

Fred Olver

halfway across the country. This is also true for those of us with vision limitations as well.

First of all you have to decide whether you want to continue to make use of your computer and second, how important is that access to you. The third thing for you to decide is whether you are willing to take the next step, which is deciding to use modified software to use your computer? Are you tired of having your nose pressed to the screen to be able to read that email or those icons on the screen? If you still want access to that information then you are going to have to change your method of interpreting that data. You have two choices, large print or talking software.

If you are still able to easily make use of large print then you need a program which will modify the size of the print and icons which appear on the screen. There are at least three of these programs. I will list them here, but I will not even begin to tell you the positives and negatives of any of them. Please understand though, that the more you increase the magnification of these programs, the less room you will have on the screen. Thus, by magnifying the size of the information, you are in effect reducing the amount of information you can display on the screen at one time. Keep in mind that at least one of these programs, Zoom-Text allows for the use of speech output, so you can get a speech output back-up to what you are seeing on the screen. The programs are Big Shot, Zoom-Text and Magic.

If you are experiencing a great deal of frustration while trying to read the screen while making use of a large print/

Dealing With Vision Loss

screen magnification program then perhaps you need to decide to make use of talking software. The two most widely used packages are GW Micro's Window-Eyes or Freedom Scientific's Jaws. You might want to go to their respective web sites and download their demo programs in order to help you determine which one you might like to purchase. Both of these programs produce high quality speech output of information that will appear in print on the screen of your computer. These programs are equally good; although some people will tell you that one or the other of them works better than the other depending on the application, but on the whole, they both work equally well with standard programs like Word and Outlook or Outlook Express. Check with other users in your area to help you in making your decision or go to their respective web sites and download demo's of each and use them for a while. Again, other users can prove to be invaluable resources in assisting you in configuring your computer to best make use of either of these programs.

As to whether or not the rehabilitation agency in your state will purchase talking or large print software for you, the answer is that in most cases if the need for the software will allow you to function or continue to function in a job, the answer is yes. If the need for talking software or large print software is for home use then the answer is probably no. There is one other exception and that is if you need the software in order to complete school assignments, say for college. In that case, you may find yourself the recipient of a new computer, needed software and extra large monitor if you can justify it, again, either for school or job.

Fred Olver

If you are diligent and look on the internet you may be able to find grant programs to assist you in your purchase of needed software. Another avenue is to ask Lions clubs in your area to assist you in your purchase. The state of Missouri has a program from which one can purchase large print or talking software which will allow one to access the internet, but that program is only for residents of Missouri. You might also check to see if the NFB or ACB affiliates in your state have a low interest loan program to assist in the purchase of needed technology. Whatever you decide, or whichever software you decide to use, it's got to be a lot less frustration than sitting there wishing your vision was better so you could still use your computer.

ORIENTING YOURSELF TO A TABLE

Let's face it, when you go out to eat, you want, no, need to know where everything is, your coffee cup, silverware, etc. You can always ask for the salt or packet of sugar, but when you walk in to a restaurant, the light isn't always going to be the best for you. You may be able to get a table near the window or far away from it if you desire, but this alone doesn't insure that you will feel comfortable in a restaurant after having sustained a significant vision loss.

The first thing to do is to get to a table. If this requires you to allow someone, even the waitress to function as your guide, then do so. It's much better than tripping over chair legs or getting separated from your party, besides it can turn in to a learning experience for both you and your guide. Secondly, after seating yourself, if you are unable to see the items on the table directly in front of you, place

Dealing With Vision Loss

your hands at the edge of the table in front of you, with your fingertips on the top of the table and your hands about a body-width apart. Raise your wrists slightly and spread your fingers. Allow just the tips of your fingers to rest on the table with your fingers slightly curved up. Move your hands slowly forward. You'll probably find your plate, or napkin, or silverware, perhaps a bread plate and coffee cup and saucer. Finding these items and remembering where they are will go a long way in assisting you when you want to find your coffee cup the next time. Do not move your hands forward with fingers straight out, if you do this you may knock over a glass of water or spill a cup of coffee. Let the fronts of your fingers come in contact with the items directly in front of you on the table and then determine what they are. You'll also feel more comfortable because you won't have to ask where things are, you'll have found out on your own.

One thing which I do when I go to a restaurant is to inquire as to whether or not they have Braille menus. If you are able to read large print, you may want to ask if the restaurant has one of their menus in this format. Whether they do or not, it will make your waitress more aware that maybe they ought to think about procuring one or more of these items either in Braille, large print or both. And I ask for one each time I return to that restaurant. So, now you can't read the regular menu, does that mean you should not have access to a menu which you can read?

Fred Olver

Cutting Meat

Cutting meat can be difficult. Roast beef or ham can be more difficult, because it is so thin. Sure, some folks will say they have no difficulty cutting meat, and for some this may be true, but maybe they have been doing it for 20 years. If it's going to be uncomfortable for you, just request your server to have it cut before being brought to the table. I often ask that the fat be removed from my steaks before being served, and if I'm going to order chicken, chances are it'll be boneless and sirloin tips are very good because oftentimes they require no cutting.

If you're going to be cutting meat, try and have the short side of the item facing your stomach. That way, when you measure the width of the piece you want to cut off, you may not have to worry about the length of the piece. Most times, after you have cut off a piece, with your knife, on the far side of the fork, you may want to check with your knife to determine how wide the piece of meat is, hold the meat down with your knife, remove your fork from the meat, turn your fork 90 degrees and re-insert it one third, or one half of the way across the length of the piece of meat if you think you need to re-cut it in to smaller pieces. It may sound complicated, but after you get the hang of it, you won't even have to think about it.

SOME OTHER HINTS

When I have a salad, if it's a large salad, I ask for it in a bowl. I've been pretty lucky, I've never ended up with a salad in my lap, but experience has taught me that restaurants

Dealing With Vision Loss

don't always make salad in nice, bite-sized pieces, and don't ya just hate that leaf of lettuce underneath it all? Salt and pepper are fun items, you don't need to smell them, just pick them up. Most times you'll find that the salt is heavier simply because there is more of it in the shaker. I haven't mastered catsup pouring, or pouring salad dressing or syrup, so I ask others to do that for me.

Being independent is a wonderful thing, but knowing one's limitations is a wonderful thing as well. Allowing someone to provide you with assistance when you acknowledge the fact that you need it will allow you to feel much more comfortable and relaxed. Sometimes people will tell you where food is on your plate by using a clock to determine placement, I personally don't care much for the idea, but it makes them feel good, and some folks feel more comfortable knowing where things are on their plate before they dig in. As far as I'm concerned, I can tell with my fork or knife where things are, and mostly what they are.

One thing which is a long way from dining is bouncing a basketball. I mention this, because eventually, you may find that finding something like a glass of water is a remembered motion. If you have difficulty remembering where things are, try bouncing a basketball and see if your motion memory doesn't improve. If you can learn, remember with your body, when and where the basketball will be, when you bounce it, you may find that you are able to remember where your glass or coffee cup is the second time you reach out your hand to find it.

51

Fred Olver

Something else that becomes very important with limited vision is your point of reference. Your point of reference used to be given to you by looking around and knowing where you were in relation to other people, things like windows, counters, doorways etc. Sometimes your point of reference changed, and you were able to keep up by merely glancing around to see where you were, but this may not be the case now. Use your other senses, hearing to help you out in this area, perhaps you can hear the kitchen off to your left, perhaps that drunk at the table behind you is rather loud, and sometimes you'll have enough vision to find your way out by taking some of this information in to account. Perhaps you can hear the cash register; again, it's a clue as to where you are in relation to the exit, maybe you'll get to the point that you can memorize the way in and out of restaurants you often visit.

When web site links are not readable, let the web master know about it. He's the one to make changes with regard to accessibility.

With regard to hotel room keys, I never miss a chance to ask clerks to place a piece of tape in the lower right hand corner of the key card and only on one side of it in order that I might be able to determine which way the key card is supposed to face when inserting it in the slot to open my room door

Zenith used to manufacture VCR's with audible menus and they can sometimes be found on some of the buy and sell groups on the internet for blind folks.

Dealing With Vision Loss

ENVIRONMENTAL MODIFICATION

This is a fancy way of talking about such things as marking stoves, washers dryers etc. There are talking thermostats available, some microwave ovens do talk, check with Best Buy and Wal-Mart. The last microwave oven I purchased came from K-Mart and it has bubble-buttons on it, some with pre-sets and each number has a bubble over it so it can be easily found and it's function memorized. You can also purchase dots for placement on your own micro-wave oven from Independent Living Aids and if you don't want to do that, then just put some marks on your items with Elmer's glue or nail polish. When marking a stove, just mark the point on the dial where the temperature is and also the place where it is to be lined up with. Many washers and dryers have pointers on their dials, so it becomes fairly easy to line up this pointer with Permanent Press, etc. In the case of stoves and other appliances without dials, well, go some place else and purchase your appliance, or ask the salesman to find out if Braille overlays are available. If not, then compare notes with some of your new-found friends who are blind or visually impaired to see how they would deal with this problem.

GUIDING AND BEING GUIDED

Some sighted people choose to refer to these techniques as sighted guide techniques. Somewhere, sometime, someone decided that sighted folks were the only folks who could guide people who are blind and so they called these techniques "sighted guide" techniques. For my part, that

Fred Olver

always offended me, because I have guided many a person who was blind, being blind myself, and I find it demeaning to refer to these techniques as "sighted guide" techniques. Guiding techniques, allow a person who is blind to travel about a half step behind their guide. Most often the person offering to be a guide will walk up to the person who is blind and ask "Do you need any assistance?" Oftentimes that person may say "No," I do not, but if they say "Yes," then the person asks which arm the person would like to use. Most often the person being guided will suggest taking the person's right arm, usually I choose to ask my guides, especially if it's their first time, "which would be most comfortable for them?" The person being a guide will then position themselves on either the left or right side of the person being guided and let the person know where they are. The person being guided then takes their arm, just above the elbow, or puts their hand on the guide's shoulder. I, generally have found that to take a person's arm is a more secure form of guiding since the guide may have to move rather quickly at some point and if I have their arm it will be easier for me to maintain my position just slightly behind them because my hand will not slip off their shoulder.

Guides, it is always a good idea to let the person you are guiding know about curbs, and steps, up or down, by stopping and telling them. If you go up the first step, let the person you are guiding find that step with their cane or foot or take the rail on their right side before you continue on. This is especially true when being a guide for senior citizens. It is not necessary to put their hand on the rail, however when taking someone to a table, you can always

Dealing With Vision Loss

let them know where they are in relation to the chair and ask them if they would like you to put their hand on the back of the chair so they know where it is.

Those of you who are taken by the arm, and forcibly moved, simply raise the arm being held onto, place your hand on the wrist of the offending person, raise their wrist and take your other hand and grasp their elbow, or inform them that you do not need their assistance. I will always remember the time I was forced across an intersection. I waited until the person had left, re-crossed the intersection and went on my way. If you are the person being guided by someone, it being their first time, it is very easy to teach these techniques. Suggest to them that when going through narrow spaces like aisles in a store that they put their arm behind their back, that is, the part of the arm, below the elbow. When they tell you the aisle is getting narrow, have them bend their arm so that the portion, below the elbow is behind them, resting just above their hips, drop your hand down their arm, to their wrist, straighten your arm and walk directly behind them. When the aisle again widens, have them return their arm to their side, move your hand back up to just above their elbow and continue on. It is not necessary to hang on, tight to their arm, say for dear life, they are your guide, not your anchor. If you find your guide is walking too fast, just ask them to slow down. By the way, kids, especially enjoy being guides.

When going through a door, ask your guide to inform you which side the door will be on. When they open the door, stick out your free hand on that side to grasp it, hold the door open and proceed through it. If the door opens to your

Fred Olver

left, and you are holding on to your guides' right arm with your left hand, have them stop, remove your hand from their arm, take their arm with your right hand, that is now just above their hips swing your left hand out to the left and grab the door as they move forward. Don't make them hold the door open for you; it's practically impossible for them to do that, anyway, since they are in front of you. If you are a guide and you are guiding someone to a chair or a couch, stop in front of it, and let the person know where they are in relation to it. Is it in front of them? Is it behind them? Also, car doors can be a real problem. Allow the person to open the door themselves, that way they are more aware of where they are in relation to the car and the door.

In closing, guiding and being guided isn't difficult. If you are being guided, take the time to explain how it is done to your guide. The more comfortable you help them feel, the more they will want to be your guide the next time. If you are a guide for someone, relax, take your time and remember they won't break, all you need to do is let them know when the terrain changes or there are curbs or steps, up or down.

ORIENTATION AND MOBILITY FOR ADULTS

Orientation and Mobility is a fancy way of saying "getting around." But it's just a bit more than that. Actually there two parts, the Orientation and the Mobility. Orientation is remaining "in the know," about where you are. Actually, Orientation is kind of like not using your vision and still knowing where you are. Let's say you are in a mall, you

Dealing With Vision Loss

smell leather, and so you are now in front of the leather goods store. You smell coffee and you are in front of Starbucks. Orientation is being observant enough to know where you are but in many cases using your other senses. Being oriented doesn't mean you don't use your vision, only that you let your other senses work for you as well. If you have some usable vision and you are in a Mall, you may get out your distance monocular and read store signs or if you are on the street, you may be able to read addresses, the key is that you are remaining in control of where you are and have knowledge about it at all times.

Mobility is the actual moving around, or through space. You will find in other sections of this book that I take a pretty firm stand with regard to using a cane, even if you have some usable vision and most folks do. The thing is that for most folks their field is reduced to the point that they are seeing only a small area, so using a cane makes it easier to concentrate on the area you want to look, because those stairs won't sneak up on you, and if you find the carpet, then you may be able to know from it's placement that you are nearing the entrance or exit. Try playing a game. Go with someone to the mall or to a downtown area and use them as a guide and try and determine where you are by making use of senses other than your vision. You might just be surprised at how much information you are able to pick up using your other senses.

One thing I haven't touched on is crossing at lights. It can be a little tricky if you are not used to it, and quite frankly, these days I get just a bit leery of crossing at some of the lights in the city where I live because of the traffic

57

Fred Olver

patterns. Usually left-turn and right turn traffic go first and then the straight through traffic goes. The key is not to get too antsy and go when you are hearing traffic moving forward. Chances are that it's going to turn, so wait until you are familiar enough with the traffic pattern and then go. It's okay to accept assistance and even ask for it if you are uncomfortable crossing an intersection by yourself. In shopping areas there are usually other pedestrians crossing at lighted intersections, but don't always follow them, sometimes they aren't willing to wait for the light, so you want to make sure the light is definitely in your favor before you cross that street.

Orientation and Mobility is not really that difficult as long as you have the right tools, your cane, knowledge where you are going and how to get there. It never hurts to ask a bus driver which bus they are driving, what route, that is, and try and sit across from him, close to the front so hopefully he or she won't forget about you. If you are not able to determine which is your stop, feel free to ask the driver to let you off at the one you want and don't feel bad about doing so. If you could see well enough to make that determination you would just ring the bell, so maybe you can't, so just ask. You may actually surprise yourself when you find out how much easier getting around is than you thought it would be, take your time. If you are not sure of something, ask and remember, no one is perfect, we all get lost a time or two, and the key is to be able to find your way back to the point where you started from.

Before I move on to the next section, there are a couple items I need to speak to you about. The first one has to do

Dealing With Vision Loss

with bending over. Yes, I know, you are probably asking, "why that?" Well, the truth is that if you're functioning with limited vision and you bend at the waist you can really hurt yourself. If you are too close to a counter you could actually knock yourself out. If you're just near the edge of the counter you could put a real gash in your forehead and if you're near the corner of the counter, well, that's too painful for me to even think about. Nonetheless, when you bend over please, please, bend at the knees. If necessary, hang on to the edge of a table or counter, but DO NOT bend at the waist.

The last item has to do with not sitting on a purse, a baby, or the dog. It's called clearing your seat. Before sitting in a chair or on a couch, just take your hand and find the spot where you are going to be sitting and make sure the newspapers have been moved and the dog isn't there. I've almost sat on my cat before and although she's pretty understanding about the whole thing, one could do a lot of damage to a small cat or dog if they are in the way.

DECIDING TO USE A CANE

It used to be that whether individuals had some usable vision or not they were given a white cane upon entering a rehabilitation program and encouraged to use it, at the very least, when crossing streets. Now-a-days, I see that some professionals in the field of blindness, although they might encourage an individual to use a cane, tend to want to leave it up to the individual to decide whether or not he or she wants to do so. I know, I know, you don't want to use it. People will know you are blind if you do, and besides it gets in your

Fred Olver

way, and if you're carrying a brief case or purse.... The list of reasons for not using a cane seems endless at times. The truth is, if you are legally blind, it is in your best interests to make use of a cane. Yes, it tells people you are blind, but then they won't yell at you when you run in to them. Drivers won't be so anxious to zoom through the intersection when they see a person who is carrying a cane crossing the street, and clerks in the store won't look at you funny when you ask them where something is which just happens to be right in front of your nose. Besides, oftentimes when you are using a cane and making use of public transportation your fare is decreased because of your vision limitation. Something else to keep in mind, if you are hit and/or injured as a pedestrian while crossing a street at an intersection while using a cane, you may find that the driver of the offending car is at fault. If you are hit or injured while crossing at an intersection while not using your cane and you sue for damages, and it comes out in the trial that you are legally blind, you, not the driver might be considered to be at fault since you are considered legally blind and not using a cane. I'm a firm believer in using a cane, because it makes good sense. I learned to use my first cane when I was seventeen, and except when I was using a dog guide, I take it with me, everywhere I go. By the way, folding and telescopic canes fit nicely in to purses or pockets and don't stick out in the aisle when in restaurants. Which brings me to my next comments concerning dog guides.

YOU AND DOG GUIDES

I just can't tell you how many times I have been asked "how come you don't have a seeing eye dog?" Well, there

Dealing With Vision Loss

are lots of reasons, but the fact is, that most sighted people look at dog guides as "Wonder-dogs." When in reality, if you don't know how to get some place, how are you going to tell your dog to get you there? When you look at the list of resources in this book, you will not find any dog guide schools listed. There is a specific reason for that. Most schools which train people who are blind to make use of dog guides like those individuals to be proficient in the use of a cane, FIRST. Consequently, whether you want to use a cane or not, if you are thinking about getting a dog you need to learn to use a cane first.

My own experience has taught me that, while using a dog guide, my orientation skills, that is to say that my skills of "knowing where I was in relation to my environment" deteriorated. I was relying on my dog, as I was supposed to, so much, that I inadvertently became less aware of what was around me. Partly because I was not using my cane to be able to know that that trash can or bench was there, because my dog guide was taking me around it, as he was supposed to, but I found that when I didn't have my dog with me that getting around, maintaining my orientation and being mobile was a much more difficult proposition than with a dog and that in order for me to be able to maintain my orientation skills that I needed to stop using a dog.

Over the years, dog guide schools have modified their stand on using canes and dogs. Used to be when you would go to the school, they would take your cane away from you. Now, some schools encourage folks to use their canes in unfamiliar areas, or in order to help you to determine where you are in

Fred Olver

relation to objects around you. A footnote to these comments concerning dogs, when I was learning to use a cane, I asked my Mobility instructor whether or not I ought to consider getting a dog guide? He said "no", that my skills were good enough that I didn't need one. Turns out he was right.

BARRIERS AND OVERCOMING THEM

In speaking about barriers, one must first of all determine what those barriers are, and where they are. The second step would be to determine whether or not you want to tackle those barriers, and how to overcome them. Some battles are worth fighting and some are not. The choice is not how to overcome a particular barrier, but whether to do so. Barriers can come in several forms. There are to my knowledge, at least two types but perhaps more.

The first of these would be man made in nature. These might manifest themselves in any number of ways including:
- Distance & Transportation
- Lack of knowledge.

The second barrier is, simply put, one's self. This can be manifested in:
- Lack of education
- Lack of awareness
- Insufficient role models
- Poor self-esteem

Man Made Barriers

With regard to distance, people who are blind are probably most limited in their efforts to travel, gain employment

Dealing With Vision Loss

and live independently by the distance they must travel and the lack of transportation available to them. Society in general seems to be rather reluctant to fund community transportation, even in the larger metropolitan areas, because most people don't make use of it, they would rather go to work one person in each vehicle. Of course in small towns it becomes more difficult because in general there is little if any public transportation available. In larger metropolitan areas, there may be public transportation, however, oftentimes that utility is not available because of all of their appointments being booked, or covers only a limited area, within a very limited time frame. Imagine only being able to go to the store between 8:30 A.M. and 5:00 P.M., Monday through Friday and even more, having to know a day ahead that you will need to go to the store. In the case of a doctor's appointment, some transportation sources will allow you a few days ahead of time to make your reservation. In many cases your time slot for your return home after your appointment may be filled. You may find yourself sitting around for a couple hours until you can be picked up.

Concerning lack of knowledge. What has been your learning curve with regard to blindness? Have people who are blind been portrayed as positive role models in society, or have they been portrayed as helpless, dependent souls with little or no ability or have they been portrayed as the "super blink" able to go anywhere and do anything? Oftentimes, people's perspective is gained on false information, for example, how they would feel about or cope with a loss of vision, or the way people who are blind are portrayed in movies or in television series. So, what is your perspective

Fred Olver

on blindness? Do you know about talking software, or software, which enlarges the size of letters on the screen? Do you know that 70% of all blind people in this country are either underemployed or not employed at all?

Self-made Barriers

Now let's take a look at the other side of the coin. In my opening, I referred to them as self-made barriers, but in thinking about them, I begin to wonder whether they might be imposed upon blind people by society itself, hence societal barriers. If society in general has a limited view as to what the needs and capabilities are of people who are blind, then how can they begin to meet their needs?

1. Lack of education

This area is one of the most difficult to deal with. As stated earlier in this book, not all blind children receive the same education. Many states do not require teachers of the blind and visually impaired to have a working knowledge of Braille. Consequently, thousands of blind kids have graduated high school even though they are functionally illiterate. Secondly, sometimes school districts do not offer programs for children who are visually impaired, or the child who is blind receives a less than adequate education because school districts are unwilling to hire professionals with degrees in the fields of Orientation and Mobility, and in special education with an emphasis on teaching visually impaired children. In this case, kids who

Dealing With Vision Loss

are blind are placed in classes with children having other disabilities simply because there is no other placement for them within that particular school district.

In the case of adults receiving services through state rehabilitation agencies, there is a long history of hiring individuals without degrees in the field of rehabilitation teaching and Orientation and Mobility. I personally have worked with individuals who have received 6-weeks training in both of these areas, who have been expected to be able to teach the candidates for rehabilitation services which come through the rehabilitation agency. This saves the state agencies money, lots of it, but shortchanges the individual receiving training because he or she will probably not become competent in areas taught by sub-standard instructors, simply because the instructor does not have competence in such areas as Braille, technology or use of a cane. Another aspect is that many administrators feel that simply because a person is blind, automatically qualifies them to be an instructor or supervisor. We require lawyers, doctors, and most professionals providing direct services of a specific nature to individuals to have received degrees in those specific areas, and in some cases, certification in order to provide specialized services, so why shouldn't state agencies providing services to individuals going through the rehabilitation process require the same of its professionals? Again, this presents problems for the client of rehabilitation services because they may receive inferior training as a result of the lack of qualifications or knowledge in the field of blindness; including the needs of the individual not having received adequate training in such areas as: low vision, adjustment to blindness,

Fred Olver

assistive technology training, adaptive cooking skills, Braille, abacus and orientation and mobility. Something else to think about is the possibility that although their instructor might not be qualified to teach the individual going through the rehabilitation process, the student might not even be aware of the lack of qualifications of their instructor.

2. Lack of Awareness

One of the most important things for a person who is blind to learn is a sense of awareness concerning training programs and avenues of opportunity which are open to them. Let's say tomorrow you wake up, and you're blind. This can happen, if you have glaucoma, or diabetes. After you go through a period of depression, fighting the fact that you are blind, hoping and praying that you will get your sight back, one day you wake up, and light dawns, you want to go on with your life. Where do you go, and what do you do? So, you find out about a rehabilitation agency, you're saved but wait, what if after your training you find out about classes that weren't offered that are, you feel, essential to your being able to move forward in your life? Ah, advocacy. Why do blind folks get involved in advocacy for themselves and others like themselves? Because in many cases they become aware of other programs in other states, which may offer more options with regard to possible avenues of training. Perhaps another state will pay for students to attend computer training programs and yours won't. Maybe you worked at home with a Rehabilitation Teacher and you want to be able to attend a rehabilitation center and your counselor

Dealing With Vision Loss

won't let you. What are your options, and how do you find out? Counselors aren't always going to be straight-forward with you. They aren't always going to tell you how to buck the system which they are a part of. There may indeed be an appeals process, however because you, the person is in effect a newbie at being blind you may not know all the in's and out's of the blindness system and some state agencies are more than willing to take advantage of that fact.

On the other hand it might be something as simple as just feeling frustrated about not getting out of the rehabilitation process what you expected or feeling like the agency providing services has let you down in terms of providing the services you feel you need.

In either case, getting involved with consumer organizations like the NFB or ACB may be the answer because both of them will provide you with resources which you might not have known about and most certainly a conduit through which you can express your frustrations and perhaps have them acted upon, or find ways to act upon them yourself.

3. Insufficient role models

When I was growing up, I went to school with other kids who were blind. Some of us were lucky enough to have gone to one of the first pre-school programs in the nation for children who were blind, before going on to a school for the blind. However, one does not look to their peers as role models. One looks to athletes, movie stars, rock-n-roll singers, authors, TV personalities your teachers

Fred Olver

and neighbors etc. Think about it, you can see how your brother or sister copes with different situations; you can see how your favorite movie star dresses and wears their hair. You can see on TV how your favorite series character copes on a daily basis with every-day situations, but what about the child who is blind? To whom do they look to as role models, as examples of individuals within the community who work, take care of their families and generally speaking, function as role models for other blind folks? True, I went to a school for the blind, so I received lots of information from other kids older than me, and we did have a few teachers who were blind, but what about the kids in public schools today who are blind, who are their role models?

4. Poor self-esteem

If kids and adults who are blind are not taught to do things, or not shown how to do things for fear they might hurt themselves, how do you think that person is going to feel about themselves as they grow up, or as an adult having recently lost some or all of their vision? Imagine standing on a street corner and having someone grab your arm and forcibly taking you across the street, whether you want to cross it or not. Imagine going in to a restaurant and having the waitress speaking to your friend about you rather than to you. "What does he want?" Imagine not having access to your local newspaper, the mail that arrives in your mailbox each day and having to have other people who can see reading your bank statement. Imagine being isolated from other people, others who are, like yourself, blind, most of the time, and imagine that when you are lucky enough to

Dealing With Vision Loss

be with other blind folks that sighted folks are constantly mooning over you, not letting you do things for yourself, and when you try to do something, having them over-ride your decision simply because they think they know more about your capabilities than you do.

This is where consumer organizations of people who are blind come in to play. There are three such organizations, the NFB, BVA and the ACB. These organizations may differ in their thinking as to how to go about getting things done, but all three are basically working for the same thing, opportunity and equality for people who are blind.

The NFB, the organization with which I am most familiar has affiliates in all 50 states, the District of Columbia and Puerto Rico. The federation in many of its state affiliates has sponsored Braille Literacy laws in order that blind children may learn to read. It also offers membership in over 50 divisions such as: a student organization for high school and college students, The National Association of Blind Lawyers, National Organization of Parents of Blind Children, medical transcriptionists, teachers, writers and many, many more as well as three centers which offer training to blind and visually impaired individuals. Each year the NFB and ACB hold national conventions. These conventions offer people who are blind, perhaps thousands of them, as well as professionals in the field of blindness a chance to meet and mingle. Topics may include: digital talking books, the future of reading for the blind, America Online, the fight for inclusion, as well as demonstrations of new talking software, hardware specially adapted for use by the blind in exhibit halls where individuals can purchase

Fred Olver

anything from a portable note-taker to talking software to that needed cane or alarm clock. More important though, these conventions offer people who are blind a chance to meet and mingle with thousands of other blind people, and a chance to see how other folks do the same things they do every day. Imagine never having been to a large metropolitan hotel and getting to and from the meetings for the first time on your own. Imagine that you've never had to do that before, and how good you would feel if you could. Imagine how good it would feel not to worry that others are "watching" you. Think about what it would be like to be with 3,000 brothers and sisters, people who fight, and win the same battles you do every day, for an entire week.

Okay, so we have these barriers, how do we, all of us, overcome them? The first step is to promote public awareness. Administrators of public buildings, corporations, schools and transportation systems need to be made aware of the needs and capabilities of blind children, senior citizens and working-age blind folks. Secondly, people who are blind need to let their needs be known by participating in organizations like Lions clubs, Jaycees and other community organizations and educating their members as to the different and varied needs of blind and visually impaired individuals. Only through participation in these and other community organizations can people who are blind, as a minority expect to be dealt with fairly and consistently. This includes things like asking your bank or utility company for a statement in Braille, asking your waitress for menus in Braille or large print, and asking instructors to provide you with examinations

Dealing With Vision Loss

in accessible formats and making sure that buildings are accessible through raised numbers and Brailled numbers on the plaques outside all rooms, rest-rooms and elevators in public buildings.

One final comment. Well, maybe, more than one. Never, never forget that you are an individual. Never allow anyone to tell you that you can't do something simply because you are blind. There is an appeal process for any public agency you will come in contact with, and each agency is required to explain that appeal process to you. If you are turned down by the Social Security Administration for benefits, there is an appeal process. I personally don't recommend hiring an attorney to assist you in this process because that will, when you win in the case that you are appealing, take needed money out of your pocket. In the case of state agencies providing needed rehabilitation training, including equipment, schooling and devices for you to be able to continue to work at a job, or aids which will allow you to get a job, there is always an appeals process. If you can't get any satisfaction from or through your rehabilitation counselor then get a copy of the appeals procedure and use it to your benefit. If you feel you need more assistance and you are a member of either the ACB or the NFB then call their national office and ask to speak with an attorney to assist you in determining what avenues are open to you. Besides these organizations, there are the Equal Employment Opportunity Commission and the Civil Rights Commission, one in each state. Do not give up.

Fred Olver

TRANSITIONS

I can't begin to answer all of the questions you might have about losing vision, about blindness, how it feels, how you are going to cope, but be assured that just because you have sustained a vision loss, doesn't mean that you have to, or need to stop living, doing or participating in the same activities you did before you became blind or visually impaired. Okay, so you're holding out some hope that your vision will miraculously return, but chances are that it won't, so you might just want to at some point, think about getting on with your life. In fact, in some respects you may find that it gives you a second chance to do some of the things you wish you would have done earlier in your life. You may not do things the same way, but you will find that with practice you can do most things either with assistance or on your own, just using different methods.

By the way, if you have feelings of suicide at times, or wonder if you'll ever get through this perceived-to-be awful situation you find yourself in, the answer is yes, but don't feel you can't talk to anyone about how you are feeling. There are agencies which have counselors available for folks just like you who are having difficulty coping with blindness. And in fact, it might not be a bad idea to take the kids and your husband or wife, with you, because I bet they're having some problems accepting and dealing with their feelings, too. You might just find that by getting involved in individual/family counseling that your family gets back on track in fact may even become closer as a result of everyone getting involved in dealing with their feelings. I realize this idea may seem to be too easy of an

72

Dealing With Vision Loss

answer; however, your life has changed, and continues to change, how you deal with the changes which have and will continue to occur may determine how successful you are at coping with your loss of vision. Eventually, though, you will, with effort find that losing some portion of your vision isn't nearly as difficult to cope with as you had first thought. It's all in your attitude.

KIDS AND BLINDNESS

*Early intervention, exposure, and
meeting the world*

Dealing With Vision Loss

DETERMINING VISION LOSS

I'm not going to sit here and pretend to have all the answers for you, the parent of a child who is blind. For the most part, doctors may be able to diagnose visual impairments at an early age but often not how severe the loss is. However if your child has, for whatever reason sustained a significant amount of vision loss you should know fairly soon after the child is born. You may find that your child is not able to track the movement of an object. You may find that your child is listless when presented with colorful mobiles over his/her crib. You may find that when loud noises occur near the child that they become scared or jump, because they can't see where the noise is coming from. Your child may have difficulty focusing on objects, even finding the nipple on a bottle. If any of these circumstances present themselves over an extended period of time you need to get your child to her pediatrician for referral for a visual evaluation. This is essential, because the sooner you begin to treat and deal with the problem of vision loss, the more the impact can be minimized. Okay, so how does one significantly minimize the impact of vision loss? A fair question, for sure, but one that will take lots of patience on your part as a parent, and perhaps having to move. The surest way, the key, the most significant item to occur in a visually impaired child's life is *EXPOSURE, EXPOSURE, EXPOSURE* to absolutely everything within their environment. I can not stress, enough, this fact. Warm water, ice cubes in their hand, a feather, perfume, the smell of a rose, laying them on the grass in your front yard, placing them in the sun so that it hits them in the face. The list is endless. Look, if your child has a significant loss of vision,

Fred Olver

the most important thing you can do is to expose them to the same stimuli they would be experiencing, using their vision by utilizing their other senses, touch, hearing, smell and taste. Remember, though, we said in another section that a person gains about 90% of their information from the use of their vision? Well, as a parent, it is absolutely necessary that your child who is blind or visually impaired be exposed to every item in your house from the stand-point of using their other senses. Allow them to grasp the pipes in your basement. Hand them a spark plug and tell them what it is. Get them involved in pre-school programs for children who are blind, as young as possible, but make sure that you or your spouse goes with them to learn how to teach your child. Show them a stack of cards, a box of envelopes, an individual envelope, an empty box for them to play in, snow flakes, snowballs, water, a glass. In a sense, you are their most important teacher, so make sure that every day, every moment counts. You may have to move in order to be close to a pre-school program for kids who are blind, so, do it. If you don't, your child may pay the price.

BRAILLE AND OTHER COMMUNICATIONS SKILLS

How do you know if your child needs to learn Braille? Well, how well is he or she able to pick up printed letters on a page? Is his/her vision going to become worse over time? Can he or she easily read large print letters? Each of these questions needs to be answered, hopefully a couple years before your child begins his or her formal education in the public school or school for the blind, in order to decide

Dealing With Vision Loss

whether or not Braille needs to be the preferred method of communications for academic purposes, coupled with other avenues such as computers and other note-taking devices. If your child's eye condition is deteriorating over a significant period of time then it becomes absolutely imperative that he/she learn Braille. So, how are you going to teach Braille to your child? Maybe in working with the pre-school program for your child, you will be able to find some resources for this project. I suggest that you contact the American Printing House for the Blind and the American Foundation for the Blind for more information, and as well, the NFB and/or ACB state affiliates in order to find out about their parents' groups.

It's also a good idea to find out whether there are Special Education teachers with certification in Visual Impairment teaching children who are blind, especially Braille, as well as Orientation and Mobility instructors and other parents of blind children in your school district. These individuals can prove to be invaluable resources and advocates for your child's needs, once he or she enters the academic world. It has been my experience that parents are the most important advocate their child has, and for that reason, it is most important that you, as a parent learn as much as you can about the services which are available in your school district for your child, and what skills are necessary in order for a child to flourish in the school setting.

How important is Braille, anyway? Well, it is as important as print was to you, when you were in school. And sadly, many students have graduated high school, functionally illiterate because school districts were unwilling to hire

Fred Olver

competent teachers in this area. It is a fact, that if a child learns Braille and becomes competent in its use, that child has a much better chance of gaining and maintaining employment upon finishing school. It becomes immensely easier to study using Braille books, and notes.

Have computers eliminated the need for Braille? Not in the least. The note-taking devices which are used today are wonderful devices, but what if their batteries die, or what if you have to send it in for repair, how is your child going to continue to function while their Braille device is gone? Ah, the slate and stylus, what a wonderful device, it fits in one's pocket, is portable and can be used to make labels, take notes, Braille up a deck of cards and write down phone numbers. Of course, when I learned Braille, we as students were introduced to the Perkins Brailler first, and this is very important because it gives the student a foundation to work from when they have to learn to write backwards using a slate and stylus.

Are computers important for blind students? Of course they are, as important as computers are to students who can see. Your son or daughter needs to learn to be flexible in their forms of study. Sometimes, hopefully most of the time their books will be available in Braille, but let's face it, sometimes assignments and tests will need to be done on a computer. These skills are absolutely essential in order for the blind or visually impaired student to flourish, in fact, the sooner these skills are introduced, the better. Do I need to tell you that the more skills your child can acquire will significantly increase his chances of success in the academic world? True enough, some of these skills can be

Dealing With Vision Loss

introduced upon entering school, perhaps in place of some other areas, secondary to the learning process, however, your child will have more than enough to keep them busy just staying even with the rest of his or her sighted peers.

ORIENTATION AND MOBILITY FOR KIDS

In dealing with decisions to be made about your child who is blind, one of the toughest decisions to be made is which skills need to be learned first. O&M, Orientation and Mobility as it is called, is probably the most important skill for a child to acquire because it will allow him or her the flexibility to be able to get from one place to another and feel comfortable in doing so. Necessary skills like Braille, O&M, the ability to dress one's self, feed one's self, being toilet-trained will go a long way in determining which educational setting is best for your child.

Orientation and Mobility are actually two different skills and it is by combining these two skills that your child is able to get around. Thus the goal of the Orientation and Mobility instructor is to teach their student how to combine these skills in order to be more functional. In the case of children, these skills are immensely important because they are the groundwork skills which will allow a child to become an independent traveler. The first and most important skill is Orientation. If a child does not know where they are, in their environment and in relation to objects around them, they will be completely lost. Mobility is the actual movement from one place to another, and doing so safely. The sum of these two being Orientation and Mobility. However, before one can develop Orientation and Mobility skills they first

Fred Olver

of all as we have already pointed out, need to know where they are in relation to their environment. The question then becomes how to develop that skill.

Again, as I have already said, the child who is blind needs to learn the same concepts as a child who can see, so how do you as a parent do this? The answer is movement and example. Once your child has acquired language skills this will become significantly easier, however these concepts are indisputably more important than Orientation or Mobility themselves, because without understanding of these concepts a child who is blind will not be able to move forward, through the Orientation and Mobility process.

Body Concepts

Being an adult we take these concepts for granted. Children who can see learn these concepts using visual means to acquire the knowledge and the skills to understand these concepts. Let me bring a bit of levity to this discussion by saying that for a child who is blind, there is never "over there." That statement just doesn't do it, never, never say "over there" to a child, or for that matter, to an adult who is blind. Find more descriptive terms such as on top of the dresser, in the corner, on the floor, be descriptive in pointing out where something is. Back to concepts.

So, concepts, you need to show your child who is blind about concepts like in front of, behind, beside, under, on top of. Move their body so it is in the position you want them to understand. Put them in front of the TV, behind the door, etc.

Dealing With Vision Loss

Show them how a room is laid out, or encourage them to find their way around a room. One of the best ways to have a child explore a room is by moving around the outside walls of the room and finding out where furniture such as tables, chairs and couches are located. If your child is comfortable doing so, have them move or walk across the room, from one side to another, through the center if possible. The important thing is for them to understand the concept of not having to walk all the way around the outside of a room to get from one point to another, but that they can walk through the center of the room. There is a certain amount of safety involved in teaching a child how to explore a room, an Orientation and Mobility instructor should know how to teach your child about trailing a wall and why it is important to squat rather than bend at the waist because of the possibility of striking a cupboard or table if one bends at the waist. Once the concepts of forward, backward, behind, in front of, beside, under, on top of, and others which I can't think of right now have been mastered then it is time to move on to the actual Orientation and Mobility skills training.

Learning to utilize these skills in concert is the key to being able to enhance one's independence. So, how does one become oriented to an area? By listening to what is going on around them, maybe the wind is blowing through the tree off to their left. Maybe they can hear the radio in the kitchen window, the key is for your child to learn and eventually know or understand. To actually be able to maintain knowledge of where they are in relation to what is around them and where they want to go and being able to figure out how to get there. Think about it, without your

83

Fred Olver

vision, you might have an extremely difficult time getting around, especially if you didn't know where you were in relation to anything around you. Again, though, by learning how to orient one's self to an area or room, or building and by remembering where one is can make all the difference in one's ability to get around. That's what makes the idea of concept building as a stepping stone to Orientation and Mobility training so important.

So, you are a parent and your two-year-old child needs to start getting oriented to your home. Maybe a bright-colored object over their bedroom doorway will help them, or maybe if you leave a radio on in their room will assist them in getting back there from the living room. If you are out in your backyard, maybe there is a sidewalk to the garage, or you might ask your child to clap their hands in order to hear the echo bounce off the house back to their ears. Learning to use this skill, "echo-location" is invaluable because it tells your child where they are in relation to other objects. When your child is very young, say two or three and you go to visit another family; you might want to take a few minutes to assist your child in orienting themselves to the area where they will be playing. You might want to show them where the coffee table is, or the TV, or the bathroom and where you might be in relation to where they are in case they may need to get to you. Remember, your child may not be able to see you, so take the extra time so they can feel more comfortable and develop/maintain their own orientation to the environment.

I'm not an O&M instructor, but I do know that incorporating sound, playing games to get a child to

Dealing With Vision Loss

move from one place to another can be a fun way to get children who are blind to feel more comfortable in their environment. Perhaps just getting him or her to bounce a ball can make all the difference in the world because it can teach remembered motion and coordination. Again, you as a parent need to take extra time with your child who is blind. You need to teach him or her where he/she is in his/her environment. Where is his/her front, his/her back, what is up, down, summersaults, how to jump, floating in the water in a life jacket, again, *EXPOSURE* is the key. Anything that you can think of which will allow your child to feel more comfortable in his/her environment and learning and knowing where they are and being able to maintain that grasp on their environment will go a very long way in allowing him/her to travel safely, efficiently and comfortably and being confident in knowing how to use his/her remaining senses to determine where he/she is and how to get to where he/she wants to be.

Encourage your child to go outside in the backyard, hopefully fenced. Teach him/her to clap his/her hands to use sound as a key to determine where they are. Teach him/her how to use reference points like the TV, or his/her bedroom in getting around the house. Bottom line, it is important to get a cane in to the hands of your blind child probably just beyond the age of three years old. I suggest you not wait until your child gets in to school in order to begin learning this most important skill because the sooner your child learns to use a cane, the more accepting of it, the more comfortable with using it, and as well, a better traveler they will become. Also, because he/she is using a cane, they will be more interested in exploring a

Fred Olver

room because they will feel more comfortable doing so. They will be able to use their cane to find objects in front of them, with it thus maintaining their orientation to new and different environments and off-setting the possibility of getting hurt by running in to that table or tripping over the end of the couch.

PUBLIC SCHOOL OR SCHOOL FOR THE BLIND

If you read the Forward to this book, you know that when I was growing up most kids who were blind were sent to schools for the blind. The reason for this was that it was felt that schools for the blind offered the best possible chance for kids who were blind, or multi-handicapped and blind to learn necessary skills. That belief has been modified over the years, so that kids who are blind are supposed to be placed in the "least restrictive environment" in order to receive their education. It is generally considered to be up to the parents of the child and the school district to decide what environment is best for the child who is blind. Of course there are pro's and con's to both, however, this is my book, so I think I am allowed to express my opinion on this matter. If your child is merely blind, I would opt for the public school situation when ever possible. I say this, because assimilation in to society in general needs to be the ultimate goal for the child, once he or she is grown. In order for this to happen, your child needs to be integrated in to the public school setting, totally. This means that your child ought not be placed in a classroom where only disabled children are present. Your child can and needs to be receiving training in blindness skills such as Braille, Orientation and Mobility, and computer skills, preferably

Dealing With Vision Loss

before attending public school if possible. After all, many sighted children learn to write and read and have some computer skills before they start school, why not your blind or visually impaired child? Your child who is blind or visually impaired also needs the interaction with other children who are not blind or visually impaired as much as possible in order to learn what is expected of him or her and how to relate to other non-handicapped children.

What if I have to move to provide my child who is blind the best possible education? My response is, why not? We are talking about educating a child which is part of a group of individuals in which there is only a 30% possibility of employment at the present time for kids who complete their education. Why wouldn't you want to present your child with the best possible chance for success in life and employment, the best possible chance to learn to be able to take care of him/herself and too, as an adult become a tax payer rather than a tax taker. I can't stress enough to you, the parent of your child who is blind how important your child's education is, and how important it is to start that education at the earliest possible moment. If you have to move to allow your child and you, or your spouse to attend a pre-school program for kids who are blind, then do it. If you need to move to a larger city because the school districts there have hired Special Education teachers with certification in teaching visually impaired kids and O&M instructors, why wouldn't you do it? You are an adult, you do have or can call on a myriad of skills in order to gain employment, and if you can't, than you may be able to find training programs in the city you want to move to which will allow you to make enough money to support

Fred Olver

your family. Your child who is blind is at enough of a disadvantage; don't make it worse by allowing him or her to languish in a less than adequate program in order to further your own career.

What if my child has other handicapping conditions besides blindness? In my mind, most public school districts have a difficult enough time dealing with kids who are merely blind. If you are lucky enough to be dealing with a teacher or teachers who are certified in visual impairment, they most certainly have taken courses on dealing with multi-handicapped children. I do think, though, that because most schools for the blind have better facilities than many public schools because they receive more state funding, and because most schools for the blind require their teachers providing services to blind and multi-handicapped students to be certified in the area of visual impairment, or at the very least, special education, that a child who has multiple handicaps is better off attending a school for the blind. This is not to say that kids who have more than one disabling condition can't function in a public school setting, only that it may be more difficult for them because they may not possess the necessary skills to be able to do their work, get from class to class and interact with other students. This does not mean that they can't acquire these necessary skills, only that it may take longer in a public school setting than it might in a school for the blind.

Ideally, it would be nice if kids who were blind could attend pre-school programs at a school for the blind. That parents would or could move to the city where the school for the blind is, so they could learn how to teach their child who is

Dealing With Vision Loss

blind, in order to reinforce what was learned during the day in their pre-school program, at home, and that when and if, the student who is blind has met specific objectives in Orientation and Mobility and Braille or large print would they be allowed to attend public schools. My perception of a school for the blind is that it should be a springboard into public school. It is important from the standpoint of what it can offer students because of the expertise of the staff. In the case of the student whose progress will be minimal, the school for the blind is indeed the least restrictive environment because of the needs of the child who is multi-handicapped and blind. I know, someone's going to write me and point out exceptions to this idea, but you see, it's my idea, and it has merit, because it offers kids who have major, major handicaps the opportunity to learn to function in the least restrictive environment for them to succeed, an environment where the staff is specifically trained to deal with kids with multiple handicaps where public schools may not be, especially when on top of everything else, the multi-handicapped child is blind.

SUMMER CAMPS AND YOUR CHILD

When I was growing up, there was about one summer camp for visually impaired and blind kids, and that one has closed and been sold. Now-a-days, there are lots of choices for families with children who are blind. Christian Record Services on their web site lists camps for kids who are blind. The state of Michigan offers access to a wonderful summer program for children who are blind, listed in the resources section of this book, Camp Tuhsmeheta with the staff themselves being mostly blind or visually impaired.

Fred Olver

The NFB also offers summer programs for children who are blind at each of its three centers in Colorado, Minnesota and Louisiana. An alternative, one which I strongly recommend, is that you and your family consider attending a national convention of either the NFB or the ACB. Their conventions are held near the end of June, or the first week in July with thousands in attendance. Both organizations have exhibit halls with information and displays of software, hardware, aids and appliances for use by blind and visually impaired children and adults and stimulating activities for the entire family. Attending one of these conventions may be the best thing you could do for both you and your child, because you will be exposed to so many very interesting people: role models for your child, the possibility of networking with other parents and professionals in the field of blindness, perhaps other individuals who are blind from your own community and information not to be found anywhere else. I know many families who make national conventions their vacation each year, because being there is so much fun for everyone concerned.

FINISHING TOUCHES

Well, that's most of what I have to say. Can you tell that I enjoyed putting this together? And this is only the halfway point. What follows is an excellent resource section with lots and lots of worthwhile resources Whether you are looking for large print books, playing cards, a cane or information about large print or talking software for your computer you will be able to find it in the resource list.

Dealing With Vision Loss

The last piece in this book is an article I wrote several years ago but never published. It is my gift to you for having purchased and read this book. It's not that the article doesn't have anything to do with blindness; in fact the opposite is true. It has everything to do with blindness because it allows you, the reader, to be able to perceive things the way I did without using my vision.

I think you'll agree, there's a lot of information in this book, not just the resources, either. Whether you are an individual who is learning how to cope with a loss of vision, their brother or sister or the parent of a child who is blind or severely visually impaired, you can't help but be affected by going through or being next to the person experiencing the loss. Dealing with a severe loss of vision isn't easy for anyone, not the family member, the individual going through it themselves or the parent of a child who is blind. Believe it or not, my parents told me that they actually lost friends when their friends found out I was a blind child, I guess their friends just couldn't cope. There's the fear factor, because no one, no one knows the exact words to say to anyone who's going through the process of losing their vision. One reason for that is that a person whose brother or mom or sister is losing their vision is complicated by their own feelings about blindness and how they might cope, or not. "Is my brother going to have to rely on me, more, to the point where I won't be able to deal with it? Is my Mom going to need to move somewhere else, and how is she going to pay for it, if she does? How do I feel about blindness myself, and how are my feelings going to affect what I say and how I react to my child, my friend or my mom?" The questions are endless because you don't have

Fred Olver

the answers, and quite honestly, no one else does either. No one knows how much vision you or your mom will lose. No one knows how you feel about blindness except you, but I can tell you this, if I were losing much of my vision in my 20's, 30's, 40's or later in life, I'd be scared to death, for a while anyway, and please, don't forget, that the whole acceptance thing is part of the process of learning to live with limited vision. One isn't going to learn that they are losing their vision one day and check in to a rehabilitation center the next day for training. For that whole process to begin can take anywhere from twelve months to two years.

When I started to put this book together, I thought it would be easy, and yes, it was easy enough to decide what sections needed to be included. When I started writing, though, I had to take a deep look at myself and determine how I felt about some of this stuff, on the inside. My sister told me, "You make it look easy." It isn't. But somewhere down the line, I had to make a decision. I had to make a choice as to whether or not I would let the fact that I was blind be my life, that is, let the blindness be the ultimate factor in determining how I would get about or through my life, or would I make an effort to overcome the circumstance of being blind and try to do absolutely as much as I can, to experience as much as I can, and to convince others that they can, too.

Sometimes I don't have much patience with folks who say they can't, because when they say that, they are limiting themselves, in their experiences and in their abilities. What

Dealing With Vision Loss

they are saying is that they don't want to, more than saying they can't. I truly believe that, too.

I sometimes find it difficult to remain patient with people who have all of their sight, and don't stretch themselves. Sometimes I even resent it because I have to stretch myself every day. Being blind isn't easy. Being unemployed isn't easy, living on disability payments isn't easy. But writing this book and developing a business on the internet is how I'm endeavoring to change my life, and the momentum is growing. I'm not going to stop trying. I'm not going to let anyone tell me I can't. When I was in sports in high school, a coach told me, and I remember it to this day and say it to myself every once in a while, "can't never did anything, can did."

I didn't think I had a book in me for a long time, even though others did. But more than that, I wasn't ready to accept the possibility of success. Think about that. There are lots of reasons for my feeling this way, or I'd like to think there are, but the truth is the reason for my feeling a lack of success is probably related to how I felt about myself. I'd like to say that it is because of the way others have felt about me, but the truth is, that most of the time, I've received pretty positive strokes from people I've met.

I will say, generally speaking, though, that most people's feelings about blindness and blind people are colored by their perceptions about what it would be like for them if they lost most of their vision. You have to keep that in mind when dealing with people. You need to realize that

Fred Olver

they have no concept of what it is like, or what it would be like for them. They don't understand that I can do most of the things they do using my other senses. No, I don't count steps; I can hear the wall in front of me. I can hear doorways as I walk down the street along the front of a building line. With the proper contrasts in environmental lighting and colors an individual can learn to get around as well as anyone else. It's when those contrasting changes are not taken in to account; it is when there are no Braille numbers on elevators or on hotel room doors that I run in to problems.

I remember when I was working on my Master's degree. I had a statistics class to take. Well, there were no talking computers, and the only way I knew whether or not I had accessed the university's computer was by how long the printer ran. No atomic science, just observation. Your senses don't get any better; you just learn how to rely on them. I'm not super, I just learned how to cope, and I hope you, or your child or your mom learns the same thing. That's why I wrote this book, so other people would learn to deal with vision loss and that it can be done, and that it's okay to be scared, just don't let it run your life.

Don't let your being scared of how to talk to me, or anyone else who is blind rule your emotions. If you're uncomfortable, let me know it. If you've never dealt with a person who is blind before, and you are confronted with that situation, let them know it. Actually, if you do, they'll probably go out of their way to help you feel more comfortable. Relate to those of us who are blind as human beings, just like you would anyone else. Be yourself, be

Dealing With Vision Loss

open, and you'll find that I'm as understanding and as caring and as human as anyone you have ever met. My blindness or the fact that your relative is blind doesn't make us different, it makes us the same as everyone else with one exception, it causes us to be more genuine. We may, at some point ask you for some assistance, that's what makes us human, the fact that we can ask for help, because most people don't.

Have a great life. Embrace your humanness, listen, grow, change and accept, because only by accepting where you are and what is going on in your life can you begin to move forward.

RESOURCES AND CATALOGS

Dealing With Vision Loss

This is a partial list of resources and catalogs which offer services, software and otherwise useful adaptive aids, information and appliances for blind and visually impaired persons. This information may also be useful to those family members who want to find Braille playing cards, large print watches, etc. for their family members. For other sites on the web, use the key words blind, or blindness. This is a fairly exhaustive list, however, if you go to some of these sites you may find other resources not mentioned on this list.

Access Technology Institute
PO Box 215151
Sacramento, CA 95821
(916) 470-6336
FAX: (800) 986-6198
Offers training in the use of talking software to be used with Windows as well as Windows itself, and for those who wish to learn to train individuals to make use of talking software.
http://www.accesstechnologyinstitute.com

Active and Able
Toll Free: 877-229-9993
From Canada: 847-229-9992
Sells adaptive aids for vision, mobility and physically impaired individuals.
http://www.activeandable.com

Fred Olver

Adaptive Sports Association
P.O. Box 1884
 Durango, CO 81302
Winter Sports: (970) 385-2163
Summer Sports: (970) 259-0374
Administration: (970) 259-0374

The goal of ASA is to persuade physically challenged individuals that they, too can participate in sports activities. As a result of their participation, individuals are able to see changes in attitude, gradual reduction of depression and a much better self-image by meeting positive role models, enhancing socialization skills, improving body image and combating depression but by most of all participating in various sports activities including both winter and summer sports. ASA is also a member of Disabled Sports USA.
http://www.asadurango.com/

American Association of Retired Persons AARP
601 E Street, NW
Washington, DC 20049
(202) 434-2477
(888) 687-2277
Largest organization of older Americans in the United States. Offers educational programs, and information on products and services; publishes a wide range of education and consumer materials. Monday - Friday 7am – 12 midnight ET. Listen to AARP on the National Federation of the Blind's NFB-NEWSLINE®. For more information about this free service,
call (866) 504-7300
http://www.aarp.org/

Dealing With Vision Loss

American Blind Bowlers Association
Linda Keeney
320 South Gramercy Place
Apt. 205
Los Angeles CA 90020
(213) 384-9613
Ginger Rush
PO Box 17588
Raleigh, NC 27619-7588
(919) 828-0945

Since the 1940's the ABBA has enabled blind and visually impaired youths and adults to bowl alongside sighted friends and family.

Throughout the year tournaments are held in many locations in North America. On or around the Memorial Day weekend a National Tournament is held in a predetermined city; this event is open to all leagues and individuals who have chosen to sanction with the ABBA. At designated times during the year, there are Area Associations that sponsor tournaments in their geographic regions; they are the Eastern Blind Bowling Association (EBBA), Midwest Blind Bowling Association (MWBBA), Southeastern Blind Bowling Association (SBBA) and the Upstate New York Blind Bowling Association (UNYBBA). A publication called The Blind Bowler is distributed three times during the bowling season (October, January and April). Articles and other pertinent information are submitted from leagues, secretaries and individuals involved in the ABBA. The content of these articles is to inform the membership of such things as ABBA business, tournament events and standings, etc.
http://www.americanblindbowlers.com/

Fred Olver

American Council of the Blind
1155 15th Street, N.W.,
Suite 1004
Washington, D.C., 20005
(800) 424-8666
Consumer organization with affiliates in most states has special interest groups involved with nearly every facet of living and working. Offers a monthly magazine, job listings on its website and other information for blind and visually impaired persons.
http://www.acb.org

ACB Radio
For on-line radio broadcast programming especially geared to blind and visually impaired users. Offers programming concerning adaptive aids, dealing with vision loss and other streams of diverse programming, including music and old-time-radio.
http://www.acbradio.org

American Diabetes Association (ADA)
ATTN: National Call Center
1701 N. Beauregard St.
Alexandria, VA 22311-1733
(800) 342-2383
Individuals are referred to local chapters for educational materials. Membership includes discounts on publications and quarterly newsletter, Diabetes, Exchange and Lists for Meal Planning. Exchange lists are available in large print.
http://www.diabetes.org/

Dealing With Vision Loss

American Foundation for the Blind
11 Penn Plaza, Suite 300
New York, NY 10001
(212) 502-7600
(800) 232-5463
National clearinghouse on blindness. Has outreach offices around the country which provide training for agency personnel and information to families of children who are blind or visually impaired. Also publishes a magazine Journal of Visual Impairment and Blindness for professionals in the field of Blindness, a consumers' magazine, Access World. They also have available a Directory of Agencies Serving the Blind and much information related to job seeking for individuals with a vision limitation on their web site. http://www.afb.org

American Printing House for the Blind
1839 Frankfort Ave.
P.O. Box 6085
Louisville, KY 40206-0085
(502) 895-2405
(800) 223-1839
Fax: (502) 899-2274

Sells puzzles, has a database of children's textbooks, products for use by blind and visually impaired individuals including computer software, reading machines, color identifiers bold line paper, Braille maps, 4-track recorders, Braille equipment, abacuses and many more other educational aids. Catalog upon request.
http://www.aph.org

Fred Olver

Ambutech
34 DeBaets St.
Winnipeg, Manitoba Canada R2J 3S9
(800) 561-3340
Fax: (800) 267-5059
AmbuTech features superior mobility products. They offer long canes for visually impaired individuals as well as support canes for people who have problems with balance.
http://www.ambutech.com/

The Association of Blind Citizens
PO Box 246
Holbrook, MA 02343
(781) 961-1023
News and Activities Line: (781) 654-2000
Fax: (781) 961-0004
The mission of the Association of Blind Citizens (ABC) is to enhance the possibilities for education, employment and generally, to advance the cause of meeting the needs of blind and visually impaired individuals in the area. By sponsoring activities for these individuals the organization meets a vital need of the community they work with: inclusion. The ABC is a membership organization of blind/visually impaired persons, their friends and families, and other interested individuals who recognize the needs and issues affecting the blind community. Visit their site to learn much more.
http://www.blindcitizens.org

Dealing With Vision Loss

Associated Services for the Blind
919 Walnut Street
Philadelphia, PA 19107
(215) 627-0600
Fax: (215) 922-0692
Offers recorded periodicals, dozens of audio recordings and Brailed books as well as large print calendars and other services to individuals in the Philadelphia area.
http://www.asb.org

Audio Editions
(800) 231-4261
Fax: (800) 882-1840
Sells books on audio cassette and CD, in abridged and unabridged formats.
Http://www.audioeditions.com

Aurora Ministries Bible Alliance
(941) 748-3031
Fax: (941) 748-2625
Provides various versions of the Bible on cassette tapes, free of charge, to blind visually impaired and print handicapped people around the world.
http://www.auroraministries.org/

Place to buy Braille/Print cards and chocolate greeting cards.
http://www.berrypurple.com/braille.htm

Fred Olver

Blind Babies Foundation
1814 Franklin Street
11th Floor
Oakland, California 94612
(510) 446-BABY or (510) 446-2229
Fax: (510) 446-2262
Founded in 1949 in response to an epidemic of blindness among premature infants. Members of the Variety Club of Northern California saw the need for services for very young children who were blind. They developed a home-based program to keep families intact. They felt that children raised in their own homes with good family support and with training in developmental skills have the best chance to be successful in life. In 2004, BBF reached over 2,000 individuals, including children, parents, caretakers, educators and medical professionals throughout Northern and Central California. More than 30,000 individuals have benefited from their services over the past 50 years.
http://blindbabies.typepad.com/

BESTMIDI.COM
A site with some humorous material and some very good information about scripts to be used with talking software and places to have your own radio show on the internet.
http://www.bestmidi.com/

Dealing With Vision Loss

Beyond Sight
5650 S. Windemere
Littleton, CO 80120
(303) 795-6455
Fax: (303) 795-6425
Offers computers and software specifically geared to meet the needs of blind and visually impaired users. Also has available, GPS devices. Authorized Dealer or Distributor for: Humanware, Dolphin Computers, GW Micro, Magnisight, Ai Squared, Eschenbach, Optelec, and Clarity.
http://www.beyondsight.com

Bibles for the Blind and Visually Handicapped International
3228 E Rosehill Ave.
Terre Haute, IN 47805-1297
(812) 466-4899
Provides KJV Bibles to the blind and visually impaired.
http://www.biblesfortheblind.org

blindbargains.com
Great place to find technology products including computers, talking caller ID's and talking watches on the web.
http://www.blindbargains.com

Fred Olver

Blind Children's Fund

311 West Broadway Suite 1
Mt. Pleasant, Michigan 48858
(989) 779-9966
Fax: (989) 779-0015
Their goal is to provide parents and professionals information, materials, and resources that will help them successfully teach and nurture infants and children who are blind, visually and multi-impaired. As well, they hope to increase global awareness regarding the need for early and continuing intervention services for preschool children who are blind, visually or multi-impaired and to engage in activities to meet the needs of these children.
http://www.blindchildrensfund.org/

Blind Cool Tech Podcasts

A place on the net to go to find out about new products available for use by blind and visually impaired individuals. This site has an emphasis on presenting information in the format of downloadable programs which can be played on a computer MP3 player or I-Pod.
http://www.blindcooltechpodcast.com

blindkiss.com

This website offers a unique perspective, because the individuals who put it together are from the UK. This site is not for children.
http://www.blindkiss.com

Dealing With Vision Loss

Blindskills, Inc.
Box 5181
Salem, OR 97304-0181
(503) 581-4224
(800) 860-4224
Fax: (503) 581-0178

Blindskills publishes a bimonthly magazine, Dialogue, primarily written by and for blind and visually impaired people, available in five formats: large print, cassette, Braille, disk and via e-mail. Its content includes information on adapting to life with low vision, techniques of daily living, career interviews, recreation and sports, technology, tips and reviews and descriptions of new products and services designed for blind and visually impaired people. Other publications include:

- *Job Hunting Resources For People with Vision Impairments*, a handbook for visually impaired people who are seeking employment;
- *Connie's Kitchen*, a cookbook which includes many tips for low vision or blind cooks.
- *Where Do I Go From Here?* a free cassette for people who are just beginning to lose vision. The tape includes a companion piece, in print, for family or friends, which gives suggestions for assisting someone with low vision.

http://www.blindskills.com

Fred Olver

blindsoftware.com LLC
Justin Daubenmire
P.O. box 145
East Palestine, Ohio 44413
(559) 224-2436
Their products are used worldwide by blind gamers, blindness agencies, and working professionals who are visually impaired. BSC is owned and operated by Justin Daubenmire, who himself is blind. For this reason, you can rest assured that BSC serves the visually impaired community with a sincere passion. They are well-known for their companion site: http://www.bscgames.com which games include: *Pipe2, Blast Chamber, Troopanum 2, Hunter, Word Strain Volume 1, Word Strain Volume 2 and 15 Numbers.* These games are playable on a Windows-based computer and can be downloaded directly from the site or purchased on CD. Blindsoftware.com offers *Day by Day* a Professional Calendar and Appointment Software and BSC Talking Clock and Reminder System
http://www.blindsoftware.com/

Blinded Veteran's of America
477 H Street NW
Washington, D.C. 20001-2694
(202) 371-8880
http://www.bva.org/

Bookshare
Offers books which have been scanned and contributed by other users which otherwise might not be available, for those who want to read using their computer.
http://www.bookshare.org

Dealing With Vision Loss

Braille Bibles International
Box 378
Liberty, MO 64069
(800) 52-BIBLE or (800) 522-4253
Fax: (877) 822-4253
Braille Bibles International provides versions of the Bible in Braille, large print and on audio cassette. They also provide two different versions of children's Bibles in Braille. The Beginner's Bible for children under the age of 6 and The Children's Bible in 365 Stories is designed for children ages 6-12. All are free to eligible persons.
http://www.braillebibles.org

Braille Circulating Library
2700 Stuart Avenue
Richmond, VA 23220
(804) 359-3743
Material on free loan for 6 weeks
Order books in Braille: Bible Studies, Devotionals, Drama, Fiction and more..

Braille Institute of America
Los Angeles Sight Center
741 North Vermont Avenue
Los Angeles, Ca 90029
Phone: 323-663-1111

Santa Barbara Center
2031 De La Vina Street
Santa Barbara, Ca 93101
Phone: 805-682-6222
Rancho Mirage Center

Fred Olver

70-251 Ramon Road
Rancho Mirage, Ca 92270
Phone: 760-321-1111

Orange County Center
527 North Dale Avenue
Anaheim, Ca 92801
Phone: 714-821-5000

San Diego Center
4555 Executive Drive
San Diego, Ca 92121
Phone: 858-452-1111

Phone hours:
Monday - Friday, 8:30 am - 5:00 pm (PST)

This organization serves adults and children in California by providing a store for purchase of various aids and appliances, a library from which books are made available in Braille and a myriad of other services is available to both children and adults.
http://www.brailleinstitute.org

Dealing With Vision Loss

Business Publishers, Inc.
P.O. Box 17592
Baltimore, MD 21297
(800) 274-6737
Primarily geared to professionals who work with senior citizens, this organization publishes a Directory of Resources for older Americans, a guidebook listing federal and state government programs, private organizations and other organizations related to aging and blindness.
http://www.bpinews.com/

California Canes
307 San Domingo Dr.
Palm Springs, CA 92264
(866) 332-4883
Fax: (877) 428-8390
Made from carbon fiber, these five section canes purport to be more durable and longer lasting than most other conventional canes. They are lighter because they are made from carbon fiber and probably give you more information because you can use a lighter touch to gain information.
http://www.californiacanes.com

Fred Olver

Camp Tuhsmeheta
Winter Address:
PO Box 18253
Lansing MI, 48933
(517) 487-3923
Summer Address:
10500 Lincoln Lake Road
Greenville MI, 48906
George Wurtzel (Executive Director)
(517) 449-2150
Jackie Hosey (Camp Director)
(616) 835-8986

General Information or inquiries:
(866) 789-9065
Welcome! Camp Tuhsmeheta is a summer camp for blind and visually impaired children and young adults located in West Michigan, seven miles west of Greenville. Camp T is an amazing place for kids to learn, grow and thrive; however it is so much more. It is an outdoor educational facility where adventure hides around every corner. It is a place where those who are blind or visually impaired can safely participate in fun, traditional camping activities that will help prepare them for a life of independence and success. It is a place full of endless possibilities for learning experiences that will help them improve their recreational and social skills. Camp T is a place where kids gain confidence while working together with their peers, it is a place where kids are encouraged by teen mentors and successful blind adults. Most of all it is a place where kids can be kids, a place where they can leave the label of blindness behind and go beyond it to discover the endless possibilities in their lives.
http://www.campt.org

Dealing With Vision Loss

Center for Braille and Narration Production
615 Howerton Ct.
Jefferson City, MO 65103-0088
(573) 751-4249 or
(800) 592-6004
Send them print materials to get transcribed in to Braille, large print, audio tape or computer files. There is a fee per page.

The Center for the Partially Sighted
12301 Wilshire Boulevard, Suite 600
Los Angeles, CA 90025
(310) 458-3501
Since it's founding in 1978, CPS has been recognized as one of the premier low vision rehabilitation centers in the world. They feel that by providing vision enhancement through the use of magnifiers and emotional support that they can assist individuals who may have sustained significant vision loss by teaching them how to make maximum use of their remaining vision.
http://www.low-vision.org/

Challenge Aspen
Post Office Box M
Aspen, Colorado 81612
Call/TTY: (970) 923.0578
Fax: (970) 923.7338
The aim of Challenge Aspen is to expose physically disabled individuals to new adventures in the areas of recreation and life challenging experiences. It is hoped that by challenging these individuals' stamina, courage and self-esteem that they will as a result grow in other areas of their lives.
http://www.challengeaspen.com/

Fred Olver

Council for Exceptional Children
1110 North Glebe Road, Suite 300,
Arlington, VA 22201
Voice phone: (703) 620-3660
TTY: (866) 915-5000
Fax: (703) 264-9494
(800) 224-6830

The Council for Exceptional Children is the largest international professional organization dedicated to improving educational outcomes for individuals with exceptionalities, students with disabilities, and/or the gifted. The Council for Exceptional Children advocates for appropriate governmental policies, sets professional standards, provides continual professional development, advocates for newly and historically underserved individuals with exceptionalities, and helps professionals obtain conditions and resources necessary for effective professional practice. Services provided include: professional development opportunities and resources; journals and newsletters with information on new research findings; classroom practices that work; federal legislation, and policies; conventions and conferences and Special Education publications. Their audience is anyone who is served by their organization and anyone who is a parent, or a professional in the field of Special Education: Teachers, administrators, students, parents, paraprofessionals, or related support service providers.
http://www.cec.sped.org

Dealing With Vision Loss

Council of Families with Visual Impairment
c/o American Council of the Blind
1155 15th Street, NW, Suite 1004
Washington, DC 20005
(202) 467-5081
Fax: (202) 467-5085
(800) 424-8666

Provides support and information for parents of blind and visually impaired children, holds an annual conference as part of the ACB convention and publishes a newsletter for parents of children who are blind.
http://www.acb.org

Courage Center
(866) 426-3442
Offers rehabilitation to physically challenged individuals and information for blind ham operators which will allow them to remain active in their hobby. Also offers training classes for individuals who wish to upgrade their ham radio licenses or receive their first license through home study courses.
http://www.handiham.org

Fred Olver

Christian Record Services
4444 South 52nd Street
Lincoln, NE 68506
(402) 488-0981
(866) 488-0981
Fax: (402) 488-7582

Provides free Christian publications and programs for persons with visual impairments. Has books to loan and Bible studies and religious periodicals free for visually impaired persons. Not all items available in all formats. They also have a lending library available for individuals of all ages and offer camp experiences for blind children throughout the United States and their families.
http://www.christianrecord.org

Canadian National Institute for the Blind
This site is available in both English and French. It provides instruction and rehabilitative services and recreational activities for Canadian citizens throughout the country, as well their site provides a host of information and related links.
http://www.cnib.ca

Crestwood Communication Aids Inc.
P.O. Box 090107
Milwaukee, WI 53209-0107
(414) 352-5678
Fax: (414) 352-5679
Sells aids for physically handicapped kids and adults as well as toys for children who are blind or visually impaired with emphasis on speech impairments.
http://www.communicationaids.com

Dealing With Vision Loss

Delta Gamma Center for Children with Visual Impairments
5030 McRee
St. Louis, MO 63110
(314) 776-1300
Center which provides services to children in the St. Louis area and has produced a book, <u>Beyond the Stairs,</u> written by brothers and sisters of blind children about such topics as embarrassment, reactions of others and living with a family member who is blind.
http://www.dgckids.org.

Diabetes Self-Management
For subscription in print:
Box 52890
Boulder, CO 80322
Has an open blog with loads of information for individuals with diabetes, provides information on diabetes management including tons of recipes. Subscription to their magazine <u>Diabetes Self-Management</u>, available on cassette, through the National Federation of the Blind.
http://www.diabetesselfmanagement.com/blog/

Dolphin USA
Dolphin Computer Access Inc.
231 Clarksville Road
Suite 3
Princeton Junction, NJ 08850

(650) 348-7401
(866) 797-5921
Fax: (650) 348-7403

Fred Olver

For more than 20 years, this company has been involved in the development of talking solutions for computer users. They sell screen-reader and magnification software. The parent company is in England but has offices in the United States.
http://www.dolphinusa.com

Dolphin Computer Access Ltd.
Technology House
Blackpole Estate West
Worchester UK
WR3 8TJ

Phone: +44 (0)1905 754 577
Fax: +44 (0)1905 754 559

Dolphin has been creating software solutions for people with print and visual impairments for more than 20 years. Dolphin products have enabled their customers to enjoy the same level of independence as their sighted peers. They sell screen-reader and magnification software.
http://www.yourdolphin.com

Doubleday Large Print Customer Service Center
6550 East 30th Street
Box 6325
Indianapolis, IN 46206
(317) 541-8920
(800) 688-4442
Fax: (317) 542-6590

Sells books in large print.
http://www.doubledaylargeprint.com/doc/club_url/club_url.jhtml

Dealing With Vision Loss

Dreamtalk Interactive
This site is the home of World of Darkness, a text adventure game with sound that simulates what life is like for a blind traveler. An excellent game for a sighted person who wants to understand a bit more about what it is like to travel without vision.
http://www.geocities.com/kenwdowney/

Duxbury Systems
270 Littleton Road, Unit 6
Westford, MA 01886
(978) 692-3000
Fax: (978) 692-7912
Provides software that can produce contracted and uncontracted Braille, mathematics and technical Braille with Windows, Macintosh, DOS and UNIX programs when using a Braille printer.
Http://www.duxburysystems.com

Enrichment Audio Resource Services
1202 Lexington Avenue, Suite 316
New York, NY 10028
(800) 843-6816
Offers free cassettes, for people who are losing vision, on such topics as "the kitchen environment", "eating without embarrassment", "indoor mobility", "managing medicine" and grooming. Offers outreach programs, not exclusively for senior citizens in the New York City area.
http://www.earsforeyes.org

Fred Olver

Empowerment Zone

The motto of Empowerment Zone is "helping individuals and communities achieve self actualization and full citizenship," according to its owner, Jamal Mazrui. To the best of my knowledge and verification, Empowerment Zone has the largest public, plain text, organized collections on the following subjects: accessible education, accessible housing, accessible travel, civil rights, employment, financial advice, funding assistive technology, gender, relationships, and sexuality, health care, HTML, CGI, and Perl, independent living, Java, legal help, political action, popular applications, including Eudora, Internet Explorer, Lynx, Netscape, Notes, Pine, Word, and WordPerfect, rehabilitation, self development, Social Security, telecommunications and windows.
http://www.empowermentzone.com

Enabling Devices

385 Warburton Avenue
Hastings-on-Hudson, NY 10706
(914) 478-0960
(800) 832-8697
Fax: (914) 479-1369
Orders: (914) 478-7030

Since 1976 this company has been dedicated to providing affordable assistive and learning devices for the physically challenged and toys for Special Children
http://enablingdevices.com

Dealing With Vision Loss

Enabling Technologies
1601 NE Braille Place
Jensen Beach, Florida 34957
(772) 225-DOTS-3687
(800) 777-3687
Fax: (772) 225-3299
(800) 950-3687
Manufactures sells and supports Braille embossers. Also sells Braille translation software and reading machines.
Http://www.brailler.com

Enablemart
(888) 640-1999
Outside the US: (360) 695-4155
Fax: (360) 695-4133
Sells everything from voice-input software to modified wireless keyboards to screen enlargers and screen readers.
http://www.enablemart.com

Enhanced Vision Home Page:
Low Vision Aids, Macular Degeneration Help, Video Magnifiers & Reading Aids for the Legally Blind and those with Low Vision Conditions

In the United States:
(888) 811-3161
Fax: (714) 374-1821
In Europe: +44 (0)115 9442317
Fax: +44 (0)115 9440720

Information for people with low vision, especially macular degeneration, also sells magnifiers.
http://www.enhancedvision.com

123

Fred Olver

En-Vision America, Inc.
1845 W. Hovey Ave.
Normal, IL 61761
(309) 452-3088
(800) 890-1180
Fax: (309) 452-3643
Provides lifestyle enhancing technology solutions for those with visual or cognitive impairments. Products assist in the areas of Health Care, Independent Living, Employment and Education.
Http://www.envisionamerica.com/index.htm

Eschenbach Optik of America
904 Ethan Allen Highway
Ridgefield, CT 06877
(800) 396-3886
(203) 438-7471
Offers magnifiers for people with low vision needs.
http: //www.ESCHENBACH.com

ETO Engineering PLLC
303 Cary Pines Dr.
Cary, NC 27513
(919) 523-0205
Fax: (877) 285-7529 (toll free)
Offers accessible cell phones for blind and physically handicapped and software which will allow them to function on the internet.
http://www.etoengineering.com/

Dealing With Vision Loss

Electronic Visual Aid Specialists (EVAS)
P.O. Box 371
Westerly, RI 02891

(800) 872-3827
(401) 596-3155
Fax: (401) 596-3979
TTY: (401) 596-3500

Provides access solutions for disabled computer users.
http://www.evas.com

Exceptionalteaching.com
Is dedicated to finding and producing products that will assist: teachers of students with special needs, teachers of students with visual impairments, blind rehabilitation professionals, teachers of high school students in transition, parents, occupational therapists, orientation and mobility instructors, and classroom teachers. They offer a wide assortment of educational games and toys for teaching exceptional children. Their selections include motivational reading games, teaching aids for those with special needs and learning disabilities, living aids, products for blind individuals, and much more! You will find an assortment of Braille products and Braille curriculum including the Mangold Combined Reading and Math Program, and the SAL2 Mangold Braille Reading Program for those who wish to learn Braille. Their goal is to offer the finest exceptional teaching tools available to facilitate all of your child's or student's learning needs.
http://www.exceptionalteaching.com/

Fred Olver

for-the-people.com
From being able to play online games to classes on internet accessibility, cooking, discussions on adjusting to blindness this site is one of the most innovative on the net. You will find a wealth of friendship, support, technical assistance, educational opportunities; a variety of intriguing stores and services; many links to interesting or useful web accessible sites and programs; but most important, you're going to meet lots of other great people just like yourself.
http://www.for-the-people.com

Foundation Fighting Blindness
(Formerly National Retinitis Pigmentosa Foundation, Inc.)
11435 Cronhill Drive
Owings Mill, MD 21117-2220
(800) 683-5555
(410) 568-0150
This page includes a number of links dealing with Retinitis Pigmentosa, Macular Degeneration and other eye conditions. Also included is a chat room, and regularly scheduled chats on various eye conditions which take place there daily.
http:// www.blindness.org/forms/register.asp

Freedombox
Customer Service
(866) 202-0520
A turnkey computer system which allows the most novices of computer users to become able to make use of computer programs in order to surf the web, read email and write letters. Not only can this be done from their own computer, but from someone else's as well.
http://www.freedombox.info

Dealing With Vision Loss

Freedom for the Blind, by James Omvig
Region VI Rehabilitation Continuing Education Program. University of Arkansas, 2002. Reprinted in 2005 by National Federation of the Blind
1800 Johnson St.
Baltimore, MD 21230
This book presents alternative methods of the presentation of training for adults who have sustained a significant loss of vision. It is available from the web site of the National Federation of the Blind.
http://www.nfb.org

Freedom Scientific Blind/Low Vision Group
11800 31st Court North
St. Petersburg, FL 33716-1805
Sales: (800) 444-4443
Technical support: (727) 803-8600
Fax: (727) 803-8001
Offers large print talking software as well as hardware to provide flexibility in navigating the world of computers by offering portable devices or integrated pieces as well to work with both Braille and speech to provide speech output, large print, and the capability of scanning of letters, bills and other documents for use with Windows products.
http://www.freedomscientific.com

G.M.A. Games
Offers audible games especially for blind computer users. Also a member of the blind and visually impaired ring of web sites, a group of over 200 places on the WWW where one can go to find all kinds of information about magnifiers, audible games, rehabilitation services and places to buy specialized aids and appliances.
http://www.gmagames.com

Fred Olver

GW Micro
725 Airport North Office Park
Fort Wayne, IN 46825
(260) 489-3671
Fax: (260) 489-2608
Develops and sells talking screen readers and other adaptive products for Braille and speech use with Windows products as well as the development of an extremely small computer with speech output, the Small Talk Ultra.
http://www.gwmicro.com

Hadley School for the Blind
700 Elm Street
Winnetka, IL 60093
(800) 323-4238
Offers distance education courses free of charge through the U.S. mail or e-mail to eligible students. Courses available in intermediate, high school, university and adult levels; GED also available.
Http://www.hadley-school.org

Hear-More
P O Box 3413
Farmingdale, NY 11735
(800) 881-4327
Resources for deaf-blind individuals.
http://www.hearmore.com

Dealing With Vision Loss

Helping Hands for the Blind
20734c Devonshire St.
Chatsworth, California 91311
(818) 341-8217
(877) 422-0300

A non-profit organization whose goal is to promote social, economic and educational opportunities for the blind. Located in California, this organization is a group of blind people who want to help other blind people. It serves as a problem solving organization and is a guide that blind people can turn to in times of need. Probably the most important service offered by HHB is that of providing timely assistance to blind people in need of help. This could mean financial assistance like helping with the rent or groceries. Quite often, however, it can take other forms, such as providing legal assistance to the limits of its funds, arranging for reduced legal fees where appropriate, providing financial grants to blind students, providing mobility instruction to enhance travel abilities for blind people, establishing special programs designed specifically to meet the needs of the blind, and responding to special requests based on individual need.
http://www.helpinghands4theblind.org

Home Readers for the Blind
604 W. Hulett
Edgerton, KS 66021
(877) 814-7323

Provides commercial mail order catalogs, cookbooks and magazines in audio cassette format.
Http://www.homereaders.com

Fred Olver

Horizons for the Blind
Information line (815) 444-8800 (press four)
Enhances self-sufficiency directly by providing Braille, large print, and audio cassette instruction manuals. Also assists public and private facilities by advising on how to make facilities and services accessible
Http://www.horizons-blind.org

Howe Press at Perkins School for the Blind
175 North Beacon Street
Watertown, MA 02172
(617) 924-3490
Sells and repairs Braille writers. Also sells Braille paper and other hand-writing supplies.
http://www.perkins.org

HumanWare
175 Mason Circle
Concord, CA 94520
(800) 722-3393
Best known for their Braille Note series of portable note-takers and GPS software and hardware. Also sells accessible cell phones with speech output and blue-tooth connectivity.
http://www.humanware.com

Dealing With Vision Loss

Independent Living Aids, Inc.
P. O. Box 9022
Hicksville, NY 11802-9022
Sales: (800) 537-2118
Technical Support: (516) 937-1848
Fax: (516) 937-3906
Sells adaptive equipment for blind and visually impaired individuals including housewares, Braille paper, talking clocks, timers and large print watches, calculators and magnifiers.
http: //www.independentliving.com

Information About Diabetes
Provides information on diabetic medication, nutrition and recipes.
http://www.informationaboutdiabetes.com

Jason & Nordic Publishers
PO Box 441
Hollidaysburg PA 16648
(814) 696-2920
Fax: (814) 696-4250
These books give children much insight into what it is like to live with a disability and to be disabled. They also provide information which children from various backgrounds can discuss in very non-threatening ways. Another value of these books is that children who have disabilities may feel more comfortable discussing their disability and how they feel about it. Those without disabilities can gain a certain amount of perspective of what it is like for a child who has a disabling condition and gain much insight in to how it feels and become more understanding of the challenges kids with disabilities meet on a daily basis.
http://www.jasonandnordic.com/

Fred Olver

Jewish Braille Institute of America

110 East 30th Street
New York, NY 10016
(212) 889 2525
(800) 433-1531
Their Library provides visually impaired, blind, physically handicapped and reading disabled of all backgrounds and ages with books, magazines and cultural programs available in Audio (in 7 languages), in Large Print and in Braille. As well, JBI loans thousands of books of Jewish interest on audio cassette, in Braille and in large print free of charge to anyone who is blind, visually impaired, physically handicapped or learning disabled.
http://www.jbilibrary.org/

Juvenile Diabetes Research Foundation International

120 Wall Street, 19th Floor
New York, NY 10005
(212) 785-9500
(800) 533- 2873

JDRF is the leading advocate of Type 1 (juvenile) diabetes research worldwide. Their mission is to find a cure for diabetes and its complications through the support of research. Since its founding in 1970 JDRF has awarded more than $1 billion to diabetes research, including more than $122 million in FY2006. In FY2006, the Foundation funded 500 centers, grants and fellowships in 20 countries.
http://www.jdrf.org/

Dealing With Vision Loss

Kurzweil Educational Systems, Inc.
100 Crosby Drive
Bedford, MA 01730-1402
By phone: from the USA or Canada: (800) 894-5374
From all other countries: (781) 276-0600
Kurzweil 1000 provides blind users access to printed and electronic materials. Printed documents (after being scanned) and digital files (such as eBooks or email) are converted from text to speech and read aloud.
http://www.kurzweiledu.com

Liberty Medical
10045 South U.S. Federal Highway
Port St. Lucie, FL 34952
(800) 633-2001
(866) 691-9277
Sells diabetic supplies, talking blood glucose monitors by Johnson and Johnson and Boeringer, insulin measuring devices; which allow a blind or visually impaired person to measure out their own insulin.
http://www.libertymedical.com/

The Lighthouse International
111 East 59th Street, 12th floor
New York, NY 10022-1202

(800) 829-0500 or California 800-826-4200
Tel: (212) 821-9200
Fax: (212) 821-9707
TTY: (212) 821-9713

Fred Olver

Manhattan/Bronx/Queens/Brooklyn
Staten Island/Long Island
Tel: (212) 821-9235
Fax: (212) 821-9743

Hudson Valley Region
Westchester County
170 Hamilton Avenue
White Plains, NY 10601-1715
Tel: (914) 683-7500
Fax: (914) 686-5866

Mid-Hudson Valley
110 Main Street
Poughkeepsie, NY 12601-3083
Tel: (845) 473-2660
Fax: (845) 473-7350

http://www.visionconnection.org

To find out more about continuing education for professionals and paraprofessionals, or to register for courses
Tel: (212) 821-9470
Fax: (212) 821-9705
Premier agency in the New York City area offering rehabilitation services, low vision screening, education for those working in the field of blindness, research, prevention, advocacy and Preschool & Early Intervention
http://www.lighthouse.org

Dealing With Vision Loss

Love Publishing Company
9101 East Kenyon Avenue
Suite 2200
Denver, CO 80237
(303) 221-7333
Fax: 303-221-7444
Publisher of books for Special Education professionals and parents of children with disabilities.
http://www.lovepublishing.com/

LS&S
P.O. Box 673
Northbrook, IL 60065
(847) 919-7728
(800) 468-4789, Ext. 218
TDD/TTY: (800) 317-8533
Fax: (847) 498-2648

Sells in-home aids and appliances and low vision aids.
http://www.LSSGROUP.com

Lutheran Braille Workers
13471 California St.
P.O. Box 5000
Yucaipa, CA 92399
(800) 925-6092
(909) 795-8977

Provides free Braille and large print Christian material in over 40 languages to the blind and visually impaired, world-wide.
Http://www. lbwinc.org

Fred Olver

Macular Degeneration International
The National Eye Institute
Toll Free Helpline (800) 683-5555
The National Eye Institute offers "Know About Low Vision," a free 22-page print booklet.
http://www.maculardegeneration.org/

Matilda Ziegler Magazine
80 8th Ave. Room 1304
New York, NY 10011
(212) 242-0263
Fax: (212) 633-1601
A magazine provided world-wide in several different formats for the blind and visually impaired which offers articles they might not otherwise have access to, and a listing of used items for sale and pen pals wanted.
http://www.zieglermag.org/

The Store at Vision Community Services
Massachusetts Association for the Blind
200 Ivy Street
Brookline, MA 02446
(800) 682-9200 (MA only)
(617) 738-5110
Fax: (617) 738-1247

Serves adolescents with brain injuries, blind and visually impaired individuals and adults with developmental disabilities.
http://www.mablind.org

Dealing With Vision Loss

Maxi-aids

42 Executive Blvd.
 P.O. Box 3209
Farmingdale, NY 11735
(800) 522-6294
Fax: (631) 752-0689
TTY: (631) 752-0738
Sells products for individuals with vision impairments, totally blind and hearing impaired.
http://WWW.MAXIAIDS.COM

Microsoft

Producer of Windows and other computer software has area for persons with disabilities to browse to find keystrokes for use with various Windows products.
http://www.microsoft.com/enable

MONS International, Inc.

6595 Roswell Road #224
Atlanta, GA 30328
(800) 541-7903
(770) 551-8455
Fax: (770) 551-8460

Sells products for people with vision limitations, especially low vision products.
http://www.magnifiers.com/

Fred Olver

NanoPac, Inc.
4823 S. Sheridan Rd., Suite 302
Tulsa, OK 74145
(800) 580-6086
Fax: (918) 665-0361
Sales of adaptive hardware and software.
http://www.nanopac.com/

National Association for Parents of Children with Visual Impairments
(NAPVI)
Box 317
Watertown, MA 02272-0317
(617) 972-7441
(800) 562-6265
Fax: (617) 972-7444

Operates a national clearinghouse and support network for information, education, and referral. Has workshops and conferences for parents and helps parents get local groups started. Services available for members include: a parent matching service for parents whose children have similar eye conditions, a quarterly newsletter "Awareness" available in print and cassette, as well as legislative updates.
http://www.spedex.com/napvi/

Dealing With Vision Loss

National Association for Visually Handicapped
22 West 21st Street, 6th floor
New York, NY 11735
(212) 889-3141
(212) 255-2804
FAX: (212) 727-2931

NAVH San Francisco
507 Polk Street, Suite 420
San Francisco, CA 94102
(415) 775 NAVH (6284)
Fax: (415) 346-9593

Sells low vision aids and lends large print books.
http://www.navh.org

National Beep Baseball Association
Jeanna Weigand
5568 Boulder Crest ST.
Columbus, OH 43235
(614) 442-1444
Sponsors World Series of Beep Baseball with teams all
over the United States.
http://www.nbba.org/

Fred Olver

National Braille Press
88 St. Stephen Street
Boston MA 02115
(617) 266-6160
(800) 548-7323
Fax: (617) 437-0456

Transcribers of books on computer access, self-help, and other general interest materials. Some of these books are also made available in what is called Porta-Braille format for use with some note-taking devices. Besides many other interesting books, they publish a magazine, <u>Our Special,</u> written and edited for blind women, which covers careers, fashion, parenting, cooking, handicrafts, travel, maternity, dating, health, and more. Also has a book club for pre-school and elementary school children which offers books in print/Braille format so that parents, whether sighted or blind can read to their children, or have their children read to them.
http://www.nbp.org

Dealing With Vision Loss

National Council on the Aging
409 3rd Street, SW, Suite 200
Washington, D.C. 20024
(202) 479-1200
Ordering Publications: (800) 424-9046
Fax: (202) 479-0735

Founded in 1950, the National Council on Aging (NCOA) is dedicated to improving the health and independence of older persons and increasing their continuing contributions to communities, society, and future generations. At the heart of NCOA is a national network of more than 14,000 organizations and leaders that work to achieve their mission. NCOA's 3,800 members include senior centers, area agencies on aging, adult day service centers, and faith-based service organizations, senior housing facilities, employment services, consumer groups and leaders from academia, business and labor.

Their programs help older people to remain healthy, find jobs, discover new ways to continue to contribute to society after retirement, and take advantage of government and private benefits programs that can improve the quality of their lives. NCOA is also a national voice for both older Americans and community organizations, leading advocacy efforts on important national issues affecting seniors.
http://www.ncoa.org

Fred Olver

National Eye Institute
Information Center NEI, NIH
Building 31, Room 6A32
31 Center Drive
Bethesda, MD 20892
(301) 496-5248
Publication Distribution Center: (800) 869-2020

Collects and distributes information on prevention, detection, and treatment of eye disorders. A division of the National Institutes of Health.
http://www.nei.nih.gov/

National Family Association for Deaf-Blind
141 Middle Neck Rd.
Sands Point, NY 11050
(516) 944-8900
(800) 255-0411
Fax: (516) 944-7302

The National Family Association for Deaf-Blind (NFADB) is a non-profit, volunteer-based family association. Their philosophy is that individuals who are deaf-blind are valued members of society and are entitled to the same opportunities and choices as other members of the community. NFADB is the largest national network of families focusing on issues surrounding deaf blindness. NFADB exists to empower the voices of families of individuals who are deaf-blind and the individuals themselves to advocate for their unique needs.
http://www.NFADB.org

Dealing With Vision Loss

National Federation of the Blind
1800 Johnson Street
Baltimore, MD 21230
(410) 659-9314
Fax: (410) 685-5653
Offers Books, Aids & Appliances. Claims to be largest consumer organization, leader in the organized blind movement, with affiliates in every state and special interest groups developed on accessibility and independence in nearly all facets of work life and recreational activities. Also offers hundreds of publications related to education concerning blindness and is involved in providing training to professionals in the field of work with the blind at it's international training center in Baltimore, MD and as well trains individuals in Adjustment to Blindness Training at three centers.
http://www.nfb.org

BLIND, Incorporated
100 East 22nd Street South
Minneapolis, Minnesota 55404
(612) 872-0100
(800) 597-9558
Fax: (612) 872-9358
http://www.blindinc.org

Colorado Center for the Blind
2233 West Shepperd Avenue
Littleton, Colorado 80120
(303) 778-1130
(800) 401-4632
Fax: (303) 778-1598
http://www.cocenter.org

Fred Olver

Louisiana Center for the Blind
101 South Trenton Street
Ruston, Louisiana 71270
(318) 251-2891
(800) 234-4166
http://www.lcb-ruston.com

National Information Center for Children and Youth with Disabilities (NICHCY)
P.O. Box 1492
Washington, DC 20013-1492
(202) 884-8200 Voice/TDD
(800) 695-0285 Voice/TDD
(202) 884-8441 Fax

Clearinghouse for information about disabled children and youth to age 22. Materials are available in English and Spanish. They are the center that provides information to the nation on: disabilities in children and youth, programs and services for infants, children, and youth with disabilities, IDEA, the nation's special education law, No Child Left Behind, the nation's general education law and research-based information on effective practices for children with disabilities. Anyone can use their services: families, educators, administrators or students. Their special focus is children and youth (birth to age 22). On their Web site, you'll find an abundance of information on: specific disabilities, early intervention services for infants and toddlers, special education and related services for children in school, research on effective educational practices, resources and connections in every state, IEPs (individualized education programs), parent materials,

Dealing With Vision Loss

disability organizations, professional associations, education rights and what the law requires, transition to adult life… and much, much more!
http://www.nichcy.org/

National Institute of Diabetes and Digestive and Kidney Diseases
(NIDDK) is part of the
National Institutes of Health
(NIH), an agency of the
U.S. Department of Health and Human Services.
General inquiries may be addressed to:
Office of Communications & Public Liaison
NIDDK, NIH
Building 31. Rm 9A06
31 Center Drive, MSC 2560
Bethesda, MD 20892-2560

Diabetes is only one avenue of research for this governmental agency. However it would be one of the most up-to-date places to go for information and research related to diabetes.
http://www2.niddk.nih.gov/

National Library Service for the Blind and Physically Handicapped
1291 Taylor Street, NW
Washington, D.C. 20542
(202) 707-5100
(800) 424-8567
Housed within the headquarters of the Library of Congress it Loans Braille and recorded books/magazines, 4 track

Fred Olver

talking book players, catalogues, bibliographies, music scores and music instruction materials free by mail through a network of libraries throughout the United States. They also provide large print, Braille digital and recorded materials for it's patrons. Inquire at your local library to find the nearest library for the blind and physically handicapped which offers such magazines as Reader's Digest in large print and the New York Times Large Print Weekly, Newsweek, Sports Illustrated, magazines for children and a huge list of Braille transcribers throughout the country.

http://www.loc.gov/nls/

Noir Medical Technologies
P.O. Box 159,
South Lyon, MI 48178
(800) 521-9746
(734) 769-5565
(Fax) 734-769-1708
Sells glasses with wrap around capability, which cuts down on UV lighting problems.
http://www.noirmedical.com

OCUTECH, Inc.
(800) 326-6460
Provides optical low vision solutions (i.e., telescopic systems) for patients suffering from macular degeneration and other low vision impairments.
Http://www.ocutech.com

Dealing With Vision Loss

Optelec/Eyes for You,
6 Liberty Way,
Westford, MA 01886,
(978) 392-0707
(800) 828-1056
Sells low vision aids, speech output and Braille output devices.
http://www.optelec.com/

Optron,
P.O. Box 5454
Morton, IL 61550-5454
(888) 567-8766

PCS Games
Besides offering games that tickle your ears this site has other links to game sites accessible to blind and visually impaired gamers on the net.
http://www.pscgames.net

Perkins School for the Blind
175 North Beacon Street
Watertown, MA 02472
Phone: (617) 924-3434
Fax: (617) 926-2027
(800) 972-7671
Besides the sales and repair of the Perkins Brailler, Perkins School for the Blind produces a number of publications, workbooks and instructional tools for relatives and other caregivers of people who are blind, visually impaired, deaf-blind or who have multiple disabilities. The Perkins Panda Early Literacy Program is a compilation of materials

Fred Olver

designed to teach early literacy skills to children with visual impairments or multi-handicapped children and to help parents be more involved in their child's literacy development. It is also very appropriate for parents and grandparents with visual impairments for use with sighted grand-children.
http://www.perkins.org

Penrickton Center for Blind Children
26530 Eureka Road
Taylor, MI 48180
Local Telephone: (734) 946-7500
One of the first pre-school programs in the United States to provide Day and residential programs for blind and multi-handicapped children in the Detroit area.

Phillips Magnification
P.O. Box 438319
Chicago, IL 60643-8319
(773) 881-8581
(800) 982-0226
Distributor of magnifiers and closed circuit TV's with which one can more easily read printed materials. Some of these (CCTV's) can be connected to computers in order to enlarge the images and letters which appear on the screen.

Prevent Blindness America
211 West Wacker Drive
Suite 1700
Chicago, Illinois 60606
(847) 843-2020
(800) 331-2020

Dealing With Vision Loss

Prevent Blindness America is the nation's leading volunteer eye health and safety organization dedicated to fighting blindness and saving sight. By promoting a continuum of vision care, Prevent Blindness America touches the lives of millions of people each year. By checking the eyes of millions of children and adults each year, their vision screenings help preschoolers at risk of vision loss from lazy eye (amblyopia), and adults threatened by glaucoma and other serious vision problems.

They train and certify adult and children's vision screeners and screening instructors through the only national program of its kind, providing 20,000 vision screening personnel with the skills they need to help people in their communities.
PBA Vision Health resource Center
(800) 331-2020
http://www.preventblindness.org
http:// www.diabetes-sight.org

Recordings for the Blind and Dyslexic
20 Rozell, Rd.
Princeton, NJ 08540
(866) RFBD-585
Records books and other educational materials for both high school and college students.
http://www.rfbd.org

Resources for Rehabilitation
22 Bonad Road
Winchester, MA 01890
(781) 368-9094
Fax: (781) 368-9096

Fred Olver

Publishes Living with Low Vision: A Resource Guide for People with Sight Loss, 7th ed., a directory of services and products for people with low vision of all ages, including self-help groups, the ADA, high-tech equipment, internet resources and more.
http://www.rfr.org/

Revolution Enterprises, Inc.
12170 Dearborn Pl.
Poway, CA 92064
(800) 382-5132
(858) 679-5785
Provides graphite folding or rigid canes for the visually impaired.
http://www.advantagecanes.com

ROPARD
P.O. Box 250425
Franklin, Michigan 48025
(800) 788-2020
ROPARD is the first organization in the country dedicated to eliminating the problems of low vision and blindness in children caused by premature birth and retinal disease. Their primary goal has been the funding of clinically relevant research to understand, treat, and prevent retinopathy of prematurity and related retinal diseases. ROPARD has funded research at Oakland University's Eye Research Institute, the Mayo Clinic, and Johns Hopkins University. It has established a pediatric retinal rescue lab at William Beaumont Hospital in Royal Oak, Michigan. ROPARD research has begun to identify a genetic link between premature birth and retinal detachment. Expanding lab

Dealing With Vision Loss

facilities, exploring new therapeutic interventions and further genetic research continue to be their primary objectives. http://www.ropard.org/

Royal National Institute of the Blind
105 Judd Street
London, UK WC1H 9NE
Tel: 020 7388 1266
Help Line: 0845 766 9999
They can put individuals in touch with support services throughout Europe. Also has available a research library, low vision center, children's center and a store from which to purchase various aids and appliances for blind and visually impaired people.
http://www.rnib.org

Science Products for the Blind
Box 888
Southeastern, PA 19399
(800) 888-7400
Carries talking vendor equipment, for state rehabilitation agencies, talking cash registers, scientific and statistical calculator, talking adaptation for shop tools like micrometers etc., and other custom electronics.
http://www.scienceproducts.org

Seedlings Braille Books for Children
P.O. Box 51924
Livonia, MI 48151-5924
(734) 427-8552
(800) 777-8552
Fax: (734) 427-8552

Fred Olver

Seedlings is dedicated to increasing the opportunity for literacy of kids who make use of Braille by providing high quality, low-cost children's literature in Braille. Besides offering books in Grade II Braille, they also offer books in uncontracted Braille for toddler and pre-school picture books with the contracted Braille added to each page using clear plastic strips. English/Spanish print-and-Braille books are also available. Print-and-Braille easy-readers are made with the contracted Braille and print matched line for line, with the print just above the Braille (no pictures). Braille books: (Braille only)are intended for more independent readers (approximate ages 6-14). In addition to over 500 fiction titles, you can also find a section of poetry and a section of nonfiction books available in their catalog. Seedlings now offers E-Braille books: You can now order the electronic version of our largest, most popular books for only $10 each. Learning tools will assist the whole family in learning Braille together.

Braille shirts, totebags and jewelry: a terrific way to educate the public about Braille and to support Seedlings!

http://www.seedlings.org

Sendero Group
1118 Maple Lane
Davis, CA 95616
Phone: (530) 757-6800
Fax: (530) 757-6830
Customer service for the Freedom Box
(866) 202-0520
Over the years, Serotek has added products that allow users with varying disabilities the freedom to access computers outside their homes including use of GPS hardware and software.
http:// www.senderogroup.com

Dealing With Vision Loss

Service Club for the Blind
3719 Watson
St. Louis, MO 63109
(314) 647-3306
Sells low vision magnifiers, large print timers and watches, talking and Braille watches and games including Monopoly and Scrabble. Call for catalog.

Sighted Electronics, Inc.
69 Woodland Avenue
Westwood, NJ 07675
(201) 666-2221
(800) 666-4883
Fax: (201) 666-0159

Sighted Electronics sells Braille Displays, Braille Printers, Braille translation software that is to say, both backward and forward translation software, from print to Braille and back again. Software, CCTV's, and Magnifiers, WinBraille a true Windows driver for Braille Embossers that produces Braille from almost any windows application. Additionally, they have the El Braille Assistant, (ElBA) a Linux Based note taker/computer with a Braille display, Index Basic D or Basic S Braille Embossers as well as the Everest and 4x4 Braille Embossers. One of their products allows for the translation of Braille text back to print applications. O.B.R. software can work as a Braille copy machine when using the Index line of Braille Embossers.
http://www.sighted.com/

Fred Olver

Ski for Light, Inc.
1455 West Lake Street
Minneapolis, MN 55408
(612) 827-3232
Ski for Light is a program of cross-country skiing benefiting blind, visually-impaired, and mobility-impaired individuals and their guides
http://www.sfl.org/

SmartWay Solutions, Inc.
1309 Dealers Avenue
New Orleans, LA 70123
Phone: (504)733-5888
Fax: (504)736-9620

A Talking Thermostat That Makes Programming a SNAP!
http://www.smartwaysolutions.com/the_talking_thermostat.htm

Social Security Administration and Information
(800) 772-1213
TDD/TTY: (800) 325-0778
Administers Supplemental Security Income (SSI),a program for individuals, adults, who are blind or otherwise disabled and who have had no work history, Social Security Disability, (SSD) a program for adults who have a work history and who find themselves confronted with blindness, and general Social Security benefits for the blind, aged and disabled. Has local and regional offices nationwide. Consult your telephone directory for the office nearest you.
http://www.ssa.gov

Dealing With Vision Loss

Sound-based field guide to birds perhaps for beginning birders?
http://www.nhest.org

Speak to Me Catalog
(800) 248-9965
Provides online catalog of products to enhance the lives of the blind and visually impaired. Most if not all of them talk.
Http: speaktomecatalog.com

Sportime
One Sportime Way
Atlanta, GA 30340
(800) 444-5700
Fax: (800) 845-1535
Orders by Mail
Sportime
P.O. Box 922668
Norcross GA 30010-2668

All Other Correspondence
Sportime
3155 Northwoods Pkwy
Norcross, GA 30071
Orders and Customer Service Toll Free: (800) 283-5700
International Toll Calls: (770) 449-5700
By Fax: (800) 845-1535
International Fax: (770) 510-7290

Sportime currently distributes four catalogs, each full of unique products tailored to aid professionals in carrying

Fred Olver

out specific movement programs and accomplishing their goals. If you would like to receive a free copy of any of our catalogs, please feel free to call us at one of the numbers listed above.
http://www.sportime.com

Talking Thermostats for the Blind
TalkingThermostats.com
PO Box 27145
Golden Valley, MN 55427-0145
(800) 838-8860
(763) 591-9557
Fax: (763) 544-7166
Comfort solutions for seniors and persons who are blind, visually impaired or disabled. Announces day, time, room temperature and temperature setting
Audio instructions for setting up program are available.
Free LIFETIME WARRANTY
http://www.talkingthermostats.com/

Technologies for the Visually Impaired Inc.
9 Nolan CT.
Hauppauge, NY 11788
Voice & Fax: (631) 724-4479
(866) 689-5672
Offers an exciting array of adaptive devices, software and accessories specifically designed for use by blind or visually impaired individuals. Their diverse, product line includes: adaptive computers, reading machines, Windows access software, speech synthesizers, refreshable Braille products, voice recognition software, screen magnification software, CCTV products, Braille embossers, Braille

Dealing With Vision Loss

translation software, tactile imaging products, various accessories, customized personal computer systems, and much more. As you will discover on this Website, they offer products from a number of different manufacturers, many of them products being priced below the suggested listed retail costs offered by even the manufacturers themselves. Whether it be for school, work or play, TVI offers many ways to give the blind or visually impaired person equal access to the expanding world of technology, as well as providing a means to greater independence and self-reliance for those of all ages. They are the U.S. authorized dealers for Portset Systems Limited of England, as well as being authorized sub-dealers for Premier Assistive Technologies, Index Braille Printer Company of Sweden, Papenmeier of Germany, Repro-Tronics, Duxbury, Dancing Dots and Robotron of Australia.

http://www.tvi-web.com/

Thought Provoker: a page on the *www* which is devoted to changing attitudes about blindness within and without. The site is for individuals who are blind or visually impaired, individuals who have sustained a substantial vision loss, professionals working in the field of blindness, and anyone interested in how to deal with blind or visually impaired people. There is much information to be gleaned from this site.. The thought provoker itself is an email which you can receive and read, reflect on, and if you choose, respond to. These thought provokers come out about once a week. The site also offers an archive of previously written thought provokers and the responses received for each, there are also links to other sites and stories about people who are blind.

Fred Olver

http://www.whitsacre.info/vip/index.htm

Tom Lorimer's Whitestick Website
A refreshing site with lots of interesting links and a unique perspective since the author is in England.
http://www.whitestick.co.uk/

TFH Special Needs Toys,
4537 Gibsonia Road,
Gibsonia, PA 15044
(800) 467 6222
Fax: (724) 444 6411
they are providers of carefully selected fun products designed to help you or those in your care enjoy life, and achieve more. Use this site and their catalog to stimulate your imagination, the imagination of your children, begin programs, or reinforce encouraged behaviors, there is a lot you can achieve...while having Fun.
http://www.tfhusa.com/

Toy Industry Association
Offers a catalog, "Let's Play: A guide to Toys for Children With Special Needs"
http://www.toy-tia.org

Dealing With Vision Loss

United States Association for Blind Athletes
33 N. Institute St.
Colorado Springs, CO 80903
(719) 630-0422
Fax: (719) 630-0616
USABA trains blind and visually impaired athletes in several different sports which include: Cycling, Goalball, Judo, Powerlifting, Skiing, Swimming, Wrestling and 5-A-Side Football. While many blind and visually impaired individuals have heard about their limitations, USABA gives them the tools to experience the reality of success in sports. Since it's founding in 1976, the United States Association of Blind Athletes (USABA), a Community Based Organization of the United States Olympic Committee, has reached more than 100,000 blind individuals. The organization has emerged as more than just a world-class trainer of blind athletes, it has become a champion of the abilities of Americans who are legally blind. Although an athlete may be blind, he or she has the ability to compete alongside his or her sighted peers. In fact, USABA athletes have served as U.S. Olympic Team members and won medals against sighted competitors. As more blind athletes receive the same opportunities as their sighted peers, the day has come when a blind athlete has competed in a sighted competition - Marla Runyan qualified for the 2000 Olympic Team in the 1,500 meter race event and made the finals. She has also finished as the top American in the Boston and New York Marathons.
http://www.usaba.org/

Fred Olver

United States Blind Golf Association
3094 Shamrock St. North
Tallahassee, FL 32308
Phone/Fax: (850) 893-4511

DIRECTOR OF GOLF DEVELOPMENT
Ron Plath (Oregon)
Phone: (503) 635-3715
SENIOR RULES OFFICIAL
Tom Mirus (Florida)
Phone: (407) 348-5650

Information on INTERNATIONAL BLIND GOLF (IBGA)
Bob Andrews (Florida)
Phone: (850) 893-4511
Our hope is that through our efforts, many more individuals who deal with the loss of sight understand that they truly can play the great game of golf. Whether learning the game for the first time or attempting to play again after losing some or all of your vision, this is the right place!
Mission Statement: The United States Blind Golf Association is organized and operated for the purposes of benefiting blind and vision-impaired persons and promoting the public good through programs that advance, and increase public awareness of golf among the blind and vision-impaired throughout the United States.
http://www.blindgolf.com/

Dealing With Vision Loss

United States Braille Chess Association
Secretary, Jay Leventhal
111-20 76th Rd. Apt. 5L
Forest Hills, NY 11375
(718) 275-2209
The purpose of the United States Braille Chess Association (USBCA) is to actively encourage and assist in the promotion and advancement of correspondence and over-the-board chess among chess enthusiasts who are blind or visually impaired.
http://www.crisscrosstech.com/usbca/

U.S. Blind Horseshoe Pitchers Association
Dr. Dennis Wyant, Nat'l President
395 Baytree Drive,
Melbourne, FL 32940
(321) 757-6824
Horseshoe pitching association for blind and visually impaired individuals.
http://www.midniteringers.org/

Vanduzer Braille Productions sells Braille greeting cards for all occasions. The pictures on the cards are also described in Braille.
4903 North River Vista Drive, Tucson, AZ 85705

V.I. Guide for Parents and Teachers
Guide to internet resources for blind and visually impaired people, parents and professionals in the field of work with the blind. This site is unique in that it is the only site in this list which is linked to the blind and visually impaired ring

Fred Olver

of sites which contains over 100 sites by and for blind and visually impaired people.
http://www.viguide.com

Lists of groups for blind computer users
Good place to go to find e-mail lists for blind computer users.
http://www.hicom.net/~oedipus/blist.html

Visually Impaired Groups
Another place to find email lists for blind and visually impaired computer users.
http://bvi-groups.tripod.com/index.htm

7128.com
Nice place to go to find games which blind and sighted can play and enjoy. The entire family will enjoy the games available from this site.
http://www.7128.com

If these resources are not enough, you might go to:
http://www.yahoo.com/groups
and use the key words blind or blindness to find other email lists specifically for people who are blind.

Fred Olver
P.O. Box 43006
Maplewood, MO 63143
Email: goodfolks@charter.net

A SURPRISE BONUS
JUST FOR YOU

I wrote this article several years ago, with the intent of getting it published, after enjoying all that this day could give me, with a friend of mine who was deaf. I strongly recommend it for a day, or two, or even a week if you have the time, it was wonderful.

Dealing With Vision Loss

AN ASSAULT ON YOUR SENSES

The Christmas gifts are all put away, or put in a place where they will not be obtrusive. It's soon time for the Super Bowl and then the doldrums of February and don't forget your cousin's birthday, right after George Washington's isn't it? One of the kids has the flu and the weatherman is calling for 12 inches of snow before morning and you're wondering what to do with the kids tomorrow because you have to work and then there's that meeting after school, but you think "one of these days I'm going to take a vacation, one that I'll remember and the kids will too." So you call 1-800 BUCKEYE and ask for their information about vacationing in Ohio which you receive about five days later.

One of the kids now has a rash from Aunt Gertrude's butter beans which she sent up, canned of course. The school, well, the roof fell in, and the kids had to change to a different one, even closer than the one they were attending. So you look at the information: theme parks, water parks, zoos, old farms, museums etc. The kids have to have a look and they all agree, Cedar Point!

Upon entering the parking lot you hear the sound of whistles blowing. Looking up, you notice several people, gesticulating wildly, not only with their hands but with their bodies as well, moving as though they were robots controlled by an unseen master. The chorus of whistles produces a heady exciting feeling in all those present. Exiting your car you are immediately warmed by the

Fred Olver

instant humidity which envelops you. One is nearly dazzled by the rays of the sun as they bounce off and around the hundreds, no thousands, of cars parked in the huge area. Amid these spectral objects humans walk, no jog, to keep up with their children.

Some, in high-topped tennis shoes, seem to glide easily over the ground as though floating on a cushion of air, self-assuredly, as if they have been here before. Grandma's and mothers watch furtively the actions of their children, but not to worry, the speed limit for the last 20 miles seems to have been about 10 MPH.

As you walk toward the many entrances to the park you begin to hear a low rumble as though a hive of bees were assembled, ready to attack each with its own distinct yet same rumble as its neighbor. These so-called bees are merely buses with their air conditioners going full blast, each spewing forth a mixture of hot and distinctly foul-smelling gasses which may surprise your leg as you walk by. Within, are hundreds of people: children with their noses pressed to the windows, mothers grabbing purses and young girls unobtrusively checking their faces and hair with compacts where their extra cash is hidden. These people, after receiving last-minute instructions exit the buses to join the growing throng moving toward the park entrances.

As you enter the park, with a turn-style just for good measure, tickets are torn and your adventure begins. After all, it's only noon, and after that three-plus hour drive and

Dealing With Vision Loss

the more than half mile walk in through the parking lot how could anyone be tired?

One of the first rides you see is the Demon Drop, a rather innocuous looking critter with a steep drop which seems to take you down as well as sideways with a tremendous stop at the end. After getting perhaps a drink of something cold, or using the facilities you venture forth to wait your turn. The line moves pretty fast. You take the trip. Short, it only begins to prepare you for what is to come.

Close to it is the Raptor, your first large coaster, one which has made many a first-timer quake in their boots as they perceive the course which it must traverse and, "you must remain seated through it all," can you take it? You approach with anticipation. You believe you can take it; after all, the Demon Drop didn't make you queasy, did it?

As you seat yourself, you hear the young men boast with great bravado. Young girls sit quietly, dreading what is to come yet waiting for that rush of adrenaline as the coaster begins its first downhill out of the starting area.

With a slow but noisy climb to the top of the next hill, the gears seem to click off the seconds grinding under the weight which they must bare yet easily overcoming it to send both you and the Raptor hurtling down and around the next curve. Feeling as though you are moving both forward and sideways at the same time, you try to hold your body in one place; however the gravitational forces seem to be pulling you in several different directions at the same time. You let yourself go and seem to float easily

Fred Olver

with the coaster as it careens through whip-like turns. The wind cools the sweat on your body instantaneously, and after several more hair-pin turns, faster, slower, stop, it's done.

You remove yourself carefully from your seat; your eyes having some difficulty focusing you unsteadily stand and walk away. While thinking about what just happened, you take a break to slow things down. You gaze at the ever-increasing throng of people around you. While chatting with friends you spy a fountain, walk to it and scoop some water over your head and face. It feels good and cold. The sweat you thought had gone away while taking the ride of your life is back, just as bad as before. Now and then a cloud high up in the sky moves lazily across the sun, presenting you with only a brief respite from the heat.

As the day progresses you are mesmerized by the plethora of sounds and smells and sights within your grasp. Depending on where you are in the park you may think you hear a jet coming in for a landing, but it's only the Mantis making a low-level pass. Besides the various sounds of the coasters there is the occasional seagull and sparrows galore. You may even hear different languages being spoken over the public address system. What's more, you can watch yourself on rides immediately after, via video recording close to the exit ramps. On one ride you may feel the spray of a nearby fountain. On another, you may smell slowly barbecuing chicken or ribs and on a third you can almost taste the hotdogs with mustard just waiting for you to come and get 'em.

Dealing With Vision Loss

Some lines are so short you are able to get off one ride and immediately get back in line for yet another rush, perhaps not more than five minutes later. The same yet different thrill, each time you take on the various magnums, bugs, dragons, space craft and the largest number of roller coasters in the world. There are water rides for those who want something different and Soak City for those who just want to cool off. Nearby are camp grounds, places to eat, take a swim, relax in a hot-tub or just talk with friends.

Near 6:00 P.M., your feet are beginning to hurt, you may have some ice cream or something to drink, but nothing too heavy though is probably a good idea since you never know what might happen to you later while riding a particularly stomach-wrenching ride. Besides there are those lines for the bathrooms. You see a boy bouncing a basketball, and then another and five minutes later, another, and then you discover they're everywhere, basketballs being bounced. I wonder what they do with them while on the rides? Has anyone ever been knocked out by a basketball flying around loose on a ride?

By the time it is 8:00 you notice that the pace has picked up. There seem to be many more people in the park than when you first arrived. Most seem very animated. Some are walking fast, some running hotdogs in hand, people chomping on gum, new T-shirts over their arm. You see tired mom's with babies nearly asleep and dads not wanting to tire just yet, for there's that long drive home. Most are various shades of red or pink on their faces, the sun having done its work. Most are happy, but all will definitely be tired when the day is done. Some will come

Fred Olver

back tomorrow for yet another taste of danger, of being on the edge. Others will be afraid of admitting to liking it, yet wanting just one more taste before going back to their own special place to remember next winter when the temperature is 20 below zero and the wind is blowing the snow in to frenzied drifts.

Although tired, you will remember this day; but wait, it isn't over just yet. As you ride the Blue Streak around quarter to nine, you notice the park lights have come on. You see the sun setting, orange in the sky, you know tomorrow will be like today with a hot sun and all the pleasure one could want. As you slide through the westward curve the sun and the lake both reflect off the ride presenting you with a beautiful blue and orange picture for you to perceive for what seems to be a long period of time, in reality though, it's only for a few seconds and then gone. The picture remains, much like the spots after a flash camera explodes to light for only a tenth of a second leaving your retinas to recover slowly from the exposure.

At 9:30, you are informed of the Laser Light Show, accompanied by music and a fireworks display which will take place at 10:00 P.M., sharp in the main plaza. Those with sensitive ears are warned not to get too close to the video screens as that is where the music will be the loudest. This message reverberates through the park as though carried by an unseen messenger from speaker to speaker. You wait with anticipation and tired feet.

By now, you've slowed down. You've ridden most of the rides you wanted to, and some two or three times. Others,

Dealing With Vision Loss

most likely those who arrived later than you, move as though in a never-ending search for the ultimate ride. You stroll through the main plaza, smelling the food and have a wonderful half a chicken to eat which gets your face all dirty, but you don't care, it's dirty anyway and besides, the chicken tastes so good.

At ten, the show begins with pictures of the Detroit Red Wings and rock-n-roll music and dancing. Then it's on to the Big Ten schools and let's not forget Notre Dame. By now, you are tired. You hear the music; you perceive the lasers as streams of light. The fireworks can't be heard for all the noise which surrounds you. So, you wash your hands, take off your shoes, grab the kids and head out to the parking lot to find the one vehicle which will take you home. All you want to do is take a shower.

During your long walk through the parking lot you wonder "where is that car, anyway" and all of a sudden it sneaks up on you. You load the kids in, climb up front, get out the map and finally you are on your way home. As you look through your rear-view mirror you can see the park well-lit, the fire works going off and if you listen very carefully the music floats even out this far as a reminder of what you have experienced in your day at Cedar Point.

CPSIA information can be obtained at www.ICGtesting.com
226379LV00002B/3/A